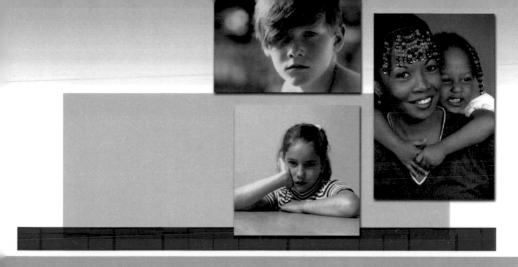

SOCIAL WORK

Seeking
Relevancy
in the
Twenty-First
Century

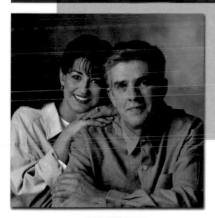

Roland Meinert

John T. Pardeck

Larry Kreuger

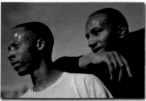

Roland Meinert, PhD
John T. Pardeck, PhD
Larry Kreuger, PhD

Social Work
Seeking Relevancy
in the Twenty-First Century

Pre-publication
REVIEWS,
COMMENTARIES,
EVALUATIONS . . .

"**S**ocial work is a profession that began in the industrial era. Despite society's transformation into a postindustrial context, social work has remained true to its roots. The result is predictable—the social work profession is losing its relevance within the current postindustrial context. How then does the profession regain its relevance and direction? Some important answers are offered in this provocative book. *Social Work: Seeking Relevancy in the Twenty-First Century* is a must-read for those scholars and practitioners looking for a way out of the conundrum."

Howard Jacob Karger, PhD
Professor
and PhD Program Director,
University of Houston,
Texas

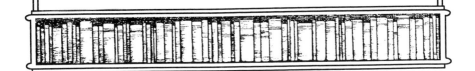

More pre-publication
REVIEWS, COMMENTARIES, EVALUATIONS . . .

"*Social Work: Seeking Relevancy in the Twenty-First Century* grapples with questions that have plagued the profession of social work throughout its history. Beginning with a question long debated, 'Is social work really a profession?', the authors move on to examine theory and knowledge, the role of research and scholarship, gender and diversity, program structure, faculty qualifications, and the role of technology. Reading this book, one is challenged to examine multiple theories and assumptions, professional stature, and the need to move beyond a national toward a global context.

It is a provocative work in its presentation of theory and the underlying assumptions. It challenges the reader to join a debate on the future of social work. The analysis examines the impact of theory and ideology on dialogue within and about the profession. At the very core is the question of who controls the dialogue. Serious concerns are raised about the impact of theories, technology, and leaders in the field currently controlling the direction, limiting the focus, trivializing knowledge, and moving the goals away from a focus on people and knowledge-building.

The authors argue for a return to humanness; construction and conversation; and learning, theory, and knowledge-building involving a broader range of discussants."

Cathryne Schmitz, PhD, ACSW
*BSW Director
and Associate Professor,
School of Social Work,
Barry University,
Miami Shores, FL*

"**A** thought-provoking work that asks the difficult questions and challenges the status quo. It forces readers to become reflective and to reexamine the basic nature, function, and structure of social work and its educational processes. A great book for graduate students as well as experienced social workers and educators. Highly recommended."

Francis K.O. Yuen, DSW, ACSW
*Associate Professor,
Division of Social Work,
California State University,
Sacramento*

Social Work
Seeking Relevancy in the Twenty-First Century

Social Work
Seeking Relevancy
in the Twenty-First Century

Roland Meinert, PhD
John T. Pardeck, PhD
Larry Kreuger, PhD

The Haworth Press
New York • London • Oxford

The Haworth Press, Inc., 10 Alice Street, Binghamton, NY 13904-1580

Material in Chapter 3 has been extracted from J. M. Jenson, M. W. Fraser, and R. E. Lewis (1991). Research training in social work doctoral programs. *Arete,* 16(1), pp. 23-38. ©1991 University of South Carolina, College of Social Work; W. M. Epstein (1992). A response to Pardeck. Thump therapy for social work journals. *Research on Social Work Practice,* 2(4), pp. 525-528, ©1991 by Sage Publications, Inc. Reprinted by permission of Sage Publications, Inc.; D. Lindsey (1999). Ensuring standards in social work research. *Research on Social Work Practice,* 9(1), pp. 115-120, ©1999 by Sage Publications, Inc. Reprinted by permission of Sage Publications, Inc.

Cover design by Monica L. Seifert.

Library of Congress Cataloging-in-Publication Data

Meinert, Roland G.
    Social work : seeking relevancy in the twenty-first century / Roland Meinert, John T. Pardeck, Larry Kreuger.
       p. cm.
    Includes bibliographical references and index.
    ISBN 0-7890-0644-8 (hc. : alk. paper)—ISBN 0-7890-1050-X (pbk. : alk. paper)
    1. Social service. I. Pardeck, John T. II. Kreuger, Larry.
HV 40.M4586   2000
362.3'2 21—dc21   99-045999
                                                                           CIP

CONTENTS

ABOUT THE AUTHORS

Roland Meinert, PhD, is President of the Missouri Association for Social Welfare in Jefferson City, Missouri. His former positions include Director of the Schools of Social Work at Michigan State University and the University of Missouri and Chair of the Department of Social Work at Southwest Missouri State University. For seven years, Dr. Meinert served as co-editor of the journal *Social Development Issues.* He is primary editor of the book *Postmodernism, Religion, and the Future of Social Work* (The Haworth Press, Inc.), the primary author of *Social Work: A Critical Analysis,* and the author of approximately thirty articles in professional journals.

John T. Pardeck, PhD, is Professor in the School of Social Work at Southwest Missouri State University in Springfield. Prior to this position, he was Chair of the Department of Social Work at Southeast Missouri State University. Dr. Pardeck is an advocate for persons with disabilities and for interpreting the Americans with Disabilities Act to both private and public sector organizations. He has written over 100 articles that have been published in professional and academic journals and has authored, co-authored, edited, or co-edited over a dozen books, including *Using Books in Clinical Social Work Practice; Reason and Rationality in Health and Human Services Delivery;* and *Postmodernism, Religion, and the Future of Social Work* (all by The Haworth Press, Inc.). Dr. Pardeck serves on the boards of several statewide social service organizations as well as on the editorial boards of several journals.

Larry W. Kreuger, PhD, is Associate Professor of Social Work at the School of Social Work at the University of Missouri at Columbia. He is a statewide leader in the study and analysis of the needs of homeless persons in Missouri and has made presentations at national and international conferences. Dr. Kreuger's articles have been published in several journals, including *Social Work, Research on Social Work Practice, Sociology and Social Welfare,* the *Journal of Independent Social Work,* the *Journal of Independent Social Work,* the *Journal of Compliance in Health Care, Health Progress,* and *American Communities for Tomorrow.*

Chapter 1

Beyond Postmodernism: The Challenge of Reconstructing the Social Work Profession

There is no single point in time about which there is agreement as to the definitive beginning of professional social work. Enough signal events took place in the late nineteenth century and the early years of the twentieth century to reasonably claim that its centennial can be marked with the beginning of the twenty-first century. Over the past 100 years the people who identify themselves as social workers, and the organizations they have established to represent their interests, have spent considerable time and effort in legitimating their claim to be a profession. As the twentieth century began, social workers felt confident that there was sufficient societal acceptance of their efforts as an emergent profession to argue that they were ready to join the ranks of medicine, law, and the ministry. A challenge to this assumption was provided by Abraham Flexner's presentation to a major social welfare conference in 1915, when he concluded that social work did not meet the essential characteristics of a major profession (Flexner, 1915). Following his presentation, and indeed up to the present time, much effort and resources as well as human, financial, and intellectual capital have been devoted to both documenting and demonstrating to other professions and citizens at large that social work does meet the criteria of a mature profession.

Now at the dawn of the twenty-first century, social work, along with several other professions, finds itself at a crossroad of many divergent paths. The signpost at this junction points down epistemological, theoretical, socio/technical, and practice directions that present potential opportunities for growth and development, as well as obstacles and challenges to continued professional status. Some think the new directions that are unfolding may lead to professional enhancement and new and innovative ways to contribute to human betterment. Others think the challenges to be encountered may be too difficult to overcome and could lead to the changed status of social work from a major to a quasi profession. Some occupations and professions, social work perhaps among them, may not be able to adapt and prosper within the turbulent new technological cyberspace environment of the next century. Irrelevancy is a real possibility for occupations that find themselves on the margins of meeting needs judged as critical by society.

Scholars and social commentators have not yet agreed upon a name to apply to the new era that the social professions are entering. There is agreement that the professions appear to be in the midst of the period called postmodernism, which has had a major impact on both the humanities and social sciences. While awaiting the arrival and societal acceptance of a label to describe the next period, it is prudent, therefore, to identify the forces and influences that are taking shape. In assessing and summing up the status of professional social work at the end of this century and the dawn of the next, there appear to be some areas of satisfaction for the profession of social work but several others of concern.

Examining social work from a historical perspective over the past century reveals that it was an emerging and quasi profession during the first three decades. This was followed by five decades of growth and development during which it approached full professional status and wider societal acceptance. However, beginning in the late 1980s, signs began to appear that the level of achievement in both practice and education was leveling off and was not as stable as had been thought. Predictions began to be made that social work practice as it had been known might be at an end, and social work education was characterized as having deep-seated problems. Indeed, some were so pessimistic about social work education that they thought it was incapable of preparing students to practice effectively for present societal demands and certainly not for emergent future trends (Bisno and Cox, 1997). Innovations and new directions in thinking are necessary to prepare practitioners for the new millennium. Past professional paradigms are being called into question and replaced without sufficient examination of their relevance to practice conditions.

This chapter examines the central issues concerning the opportunities and challenges facing social work at the beginning of the new century. In the opinion of the authors these are critical and defining issues that must be addressed if social work is to remain a viable profession as the next millennium begins. Indeed, these issues are of such a magnitude that their resolution will determine whether social work will celebrate a second centennial. With but a few exceptions it will be seen upon examination that most of the issues are not fundamentally different than those that faced the founders of the profession at the beginning of the twentieth century. The total array of issues poses a comprehensive set of theoretical, ideological, and technical challenges to be faced and opportunities to be maximized. Each of the issues is briefly stated below in the form of a question and subsequently analytically discussed in more detail:

- Can social work legitimately claim to be a mature profession when measured by both historical and contemporary criteria?
- Is the knowledge base of social work suspect because it spans extensive domains of practice that defy orderly classification?
- Is social work a captive of politicized ideologies that hinder its development and make it difficult to entertain intellectual diversity and the adoption of new and creative directions?
- Are social work values a myth?
- Has the ethnocentricity of American social work prevented it from adopting social development and other approaches found effective in other societies?
- Will uncritically embracing postmodernism, and a family of other "isms," result in long-range enfeebling consequences for the profession?
- Does social work have a significant impact on developing major social welfare policies?
- Is social work education in serious difficulty because it is epistemologically and conceptually without direction?

The manner in which these questions are addressed and the resources and effort applied to their solutions constitute a set of both challenges and opportunities for twenty-first century social work. The consequences of not addressing them include the possibility that social work will not survive as a major profession in a society characterized by postindustrial influences and hypertechnological advances. Social work can be reconstructed, but only if it is willing to recognize its weaknesses and use them as an opportunity to advance to the next level of development. The first step in this reconstruction effort should be to reexamine the extent to which it meets contemporary criteria for a major legitimate profession.

FLEXNER REVISITED

The field of social work in the early years of the twentieth century was struggling to establish legitimacy and recognition among the family of professions. There was uncertainty at the time as to what distinguished a professional from an amateur, and whether or not certain attributes could be identified setting professional activities apart from occupational ones. Approximately eighty-five years ago, Abraham Flexner (1915) gave the fledgling occupation of social work a wake-up call when he appeared by invitation before a major social work conference and asserted that it did not meet the criteria of a profession. He praised what social workers did, but was unable to conclude that social work's characteristics were at the same level as those possessed by other mature professions such as medicine and law. He viewed social work not so much as a definite field but "as an aspect of work in many fields." After examining the activities of social workers within multiple fields of functioning, he also did not provide a positive report about the training they received. His opinion was that the activities of social workers were so numerous, diverse, and unspecific that it would not be feasible to design a program of organized education. As the twenty-first century dawns, if social work were to be placed under an analytic microscope it is conceivable that Flexner's conclusions in 1915 would to some degree remain valid.

Recent approaches to the analysis of professions emphasize a model based on systems thinking (Abbott, 1988). In this perspective professions are viewed as existing in a system of occupations and professions, each of which is vying to establish and then maintain itself within an identifiable niche. As a profession functions within a niche, much of its occupational energy and resources are devoted to consolidating its position and solidifying jurisdiction over a set of functions and tasks. Thus, a profession engages in dynamic interaction and negotiation with other occupations to retain its positional niche. For most of the twentieth century, social work and other occupations were measured by a set of criteria to determine their degree of professionalism. When these criteria were applied to occupations, it was easily seen that some extreme variation existed. Some occupations possessed most of the criteria to a high degree and others hardly at all. Recent literature has tended to ignore the criteria or attribute model of measuring professionalism. It is the opinion of the authors that this model has validity and can illuminate where social work stands in the system of professions at the century's end. Not all attributes possess the same degree of saliency in assessing professionalism. Some attributes are of a first order or central to the conceptualization of professionalism and are intrinsic to the nature of a profession. Others, of a second order, are of lesser importance and are not essential attributes. A major profession would be expected to possess all the first-order attributes to a high degree, and minor or quasi professions would not possess all or would have low saliency among them. Occupations that in the judgment of the general public clearly are not professions possess many of the second-order features but lack one or more first-order ones. Among analysts of occupations there is no consensus on a finite list of professional attributes, but after reviewing the literature the authors feel those listed in Table 1.1 are highly representative of the opinions of most experts. Possession of the attributes to a high degree separates professions from numerous occupations that describe themselves as such but fall short. Table 1.1 lists the central first-order attributes and the second-order peripheral ones along with brief descriptions of their focus. A logical cohesiveness exists among the first-order attributes, which constitute a coherent corpus to which all major professions can lay claim.

Based on the first-order attributes, a profession meets a distinct and expressed need and is given legitimation, jurisdiction, and sup-

TABLE 1.1. Two Levels of Professional Attributes

FIRST ORDER

Niche—There exists a set of specific service activities that are carried out within the larger domain of logically related professions. The practitioners within the domain have exclusive jurisdiction and authority over the functions that are carried out. This authority and jurisdiction are recognized by others within the system of "professions."

Theory and Praxis—The skilled actions of practitioners rest on a foundation of theory or set of related theories. This permits the application of abstract knowledge to a range of conditions. Even though practitioner actions have practical outcomes, they emanate from a process that is essentially intellectual.

Societal Sanction—There exists societal sanction and support for activities in a specific domain (niche) of human need. This sanction manifests itself by approval for, legitimation of, and the creation of official organizational structures to provide services within the domain of need. The practitioners and the services to be delivered are seen as trustworthy by recipients.

Knowledge Development—The niche occupied by a profession provides the boundaries within which research and the development of relevant new knowledge take place. All professions to some degree "borrow" knowledge from other professions and disciplines. However, major professions provide sanction and resources and institutionalize efforts for this discovery process in support of their core activities.

Articulated Education—To achieve legitimation within a profession, the practitioners must have completed a standardized period of training. The institution or body providing the training must meet a set of quality standards articulated by an external review body. Periodic reviews must take place to ensure that the educational standards continue to be met.

Licensure—Practitioners must document that they have completed formal training in the profession and have passed standardized examinations which are universally accepted within the society that provides the sanction. Licensure examinations must be organized around the central knowledge and skills of the profession. Professionals are not permitted to practice in societally sanctioned organizations until licensure has been achieved.

SECOND ORDER

Professional Association—Professions establish official associations to provide some monitoring of internal functions and to represent the interests of practitioners to the larger society.

Code of Ethics—Professions presumably possess a set of internal values and norms expressive of their core nature and purpose. These values and norms provide the foundation for a code of ethics which is to guide ethical practitioner behavior toward clients, colleagues, and employment settings.

Altruism—It is believed that professions, with their orientation of service provision, have the power to attract persons who have characteristics motivating them toward a career focusing on service to others.

---

port by society at large. The actions by practitioners are founded on a body of theory and research that is continually updated and transmitted to those preparing for professional careers in organized programs of education. Upon entry into the profession, neophytes are tested in a standardized fashion leading to certification for practice. At the dawn of the new century it is prudent to ask to what extent social work meets the first-order attributes and whether, as claimed, it is seated firmly within the family of major professions.

For decades social work has selected as its main objective the enhancement of individual and social well-being within the contextual niche of the person in the environment. The niche is problematic for two reasons. First, it is so broad and at such a general level of abstraction that it appears to be without boundaries. In this regard the niche turns out to be not a niche at all because of the wide scope of reality that it embraces. Second, all professions to some degree deal with issues within the person-in-the-environment configuration, or the adaptation of the individual to external systems. Education, for example, focuses on the interaction and process of the student with the knowledge-learning environment. Other professions are also involved with person-in-the-environment issues, such as medicine, law, public health, and counseling. Social work's claim to this niche is a weak one. Problems are also present with the attribute of a body of systematic and articulated theory that is applied to practical issues. There is an absence of an organizing theory, or in the perspective of postmodernism, a metanarrative, from which social work practitioners can structure and organize their professional activities. Tucker (1996) frames this limitation as the absence of a problematic, or central organizing, question. This problem is best illustrated in the policy on concentrations at the graduate level in social work education. Programs have unlimited freedom to select any concentration they wish that is consistent with the purpose of social work (CSWE, 1994) and if there is a coherent theoretical foundation to support them. Given the lack of boundaries with the person-in-the-environment construct, the theories to be selected can approach infinity. Those who adhere to a postmodern perspective for social work practice argue that theory should be generated situationally and from within the language community of the client. This approach eschews a theory, or set of theories, as a foundation for the entire profession. Indeed, one social work leader argues that the application of imposed theory by practitioners represents a pernicious use of power and is unprofessional (Hartman, 1992).

It is difficult to assess the status of social work with respect to the attribute of societal sanction because there are no agreed-upon measures. Resources are allocated to a vast range of social services, but this only indicates support to meet a variety of human needs and not for the profession of social work per se. The same difficulty pertains to the attribute of knowledge development. Social workers are increasingly involved in research efforts, but there is a paucity of evidence of major discoveries such as those in medicine or the physical sciences. Nor is there evidence that the knowledge produced has made a difference in the world of practice. Perhaps the biggest deficiency in this area pertains to the mechanism and process by which professional journal editorial boards judge what shall be published. Pardeck (1992) and Epstein (1990) have provided compelling evidence that social work editorial boards do not possess the distinction and achievement levels to make informed judgments about whether journal manuscripts should be approved for publication. Since professional journals are the primary mechanism by which new information is transmitted to practitioners, it is absolutely necessary that those who judge the quality of manuscripts possess the required competence.

On the first-order attributes of articulated education and licensure, social work demonstrates some strength. The Council on Social Work Education (CSWE) now accredits over 600 programs at the baccalaureate and master's levels. Annually, about twenty programs are in the candidacy stage of the accreditation process and an equal number have plans to eventually pursue accreditation. There appears to be no end of colleges and universities who plan to initiate social work degree programs nor in the number of students who plan to major in social work. All fifty states now have either licensing or registration legislation for social workers. This achievement would have been seen as extremely difficult four decades ago. However, it is not unusual, and indeed it seems commonplace, for service providers to hire social workers who have not acquired licensure or accreditation by the national professional association. In this regard social work stands in stark contrast to medicine and law, where licensure is strongly endorsed by society at large. In the main the larger society exhibits disinterest in the issue of social work licensure.

Where, then, among the array of first-order professional attributes does social work stand? A reasonable conclusion would be that in terms of a specific niche among the helping professions, it is deficient. The same can be concluded about its possession of a relevant theory or set of theories that can be applied to practice behavior across diverse situations. These are serious deficiencies. It is stronger, but with identifiable deficiencies, in the attributes of societal sanction and the development of knowledge for practice. It matches the attributes of articulated education for practice and licensure most strongly of all.

THE STATUS OF KNOWLEDGE

Institutionalized social work is based on a conviction that it possesses a body of relevant knowledge, a set of skills that logically emanates from that body, and a definable value base. At century's end an analysis of the knowledge foundation of social work highlights some areas of concern. Associated with these is the question of whether social work is an art form if it is not based on the canons of science. If the knowledge base is suspect, and practice is an idiosyncratic expression of artful skills, it obviates the need for a foundation of organized theory or set of theories to guide practitioner behavior. The characteristics of suspect knowledge base, art versus science, and theoretical obfuscation are discussed separately.

A student in social work told one of the authors she felt "deceived" after completing graduate studies. Prior to entering school she had been told that it was necessary to complete graduate studies to acquire the knowledge to become a professional social worker. She was told, and believed, that an identifiable and confirmed body of social work knowledge existed and would be presented in the graduate program. She believed that something called "truth" existed outside the minds of persons and could be discovered and then applied in professional practice. However, upon completion of graduate studies she felt that her teachers had spent most of their time disabusing her of the belief that there are universal principles of the human condition. She felt that their main emphasis had been on alerting her to the contradictions, ambiguities, uncertainties, and chaos rather than on what is known about the commonality of human experience. As a young woman from a rural background she entered graduate studies with high regard for university professors and eagerly waited to find out what they professed and would transmit to her. Rather, in classes she experienced endless and unfocused group discussions in which her mentors were more interested in what she "felt" than what she knew. With degree in hand she eventually entered the world of practice, having been told endlessly that knowledge was a form of power that could be used in an elitist manner with clients. Her charge, therefore, as she understood it, was to deconstruct the social work knowledge base and seek out one that was subjectively constructed in local language communities. In addition, since all knowledge was to be considered relative, it could not be applied from one situation to another.

This student's observations identify but one of the concerns about the state of knowledge in social work. As argued by Edward O. Wilson (1998), the scientific method has resulted in an understanding of the physical world beyond the wildest imagination of earlier generations. According to Wilson there is a unity within the world even though upon casual observation it appears to be replete with disparate phenomena. One of the objectives of science is the ongoing attempt to discover a groundwork of explanation or set of theories to understand disparate facts. Social work's adoption of a perspective variously called systems or ecological theory has been an effort to discover this unity within the domain in which it operates. Postmodernists call these unifying theories metanarratives and take the position that they must be eliminated since they arise from the power and control of the elite scientific community. The challenge facing the field of social work is not to give up on the application of the scientific method in the social sciences in favor of the approaches of postmodernism, deconstructionism, and existentialism. In the latter approaches there is no consensual method and reality becomes the interpretive conclusions of whatever persons wish to make them. The student who described her dissatisfaction, was being exposed to as many versions of the truth as there were faculty. Thus she concluded that social work did not have an identifiable knowledge base, but that there were as many knowledge bases as there were participants in a discussion. In her view, and in the view of others, it is disingenuous to continue the fiction that a firm knowledge base exists in social work. An ironic and contradictory shift in the developmental history of social work appears to have gone unnoticed. For many decades it energetically worked to become a bona fide member of the science-based professions. Having attained some modicum of success in that quest, it is now working to dissociate itself from the methods that gained it a significant degree of professional acceptance and recognition. It also strove mightily for inclusion under the auspices of uni versities as a legitimate academic program. Since the business of universities is the development of new knowledge and its transmission, social work may find itself in jeopardy within the academic culture. This is because it is distancing itself from the established principles, canons, and approaches of science as it adopts postmodern and deconstructivist separatist positions.

More and more, social work is being seen as an art form employed to help persons achieve a higher level of social functioning. This view is consistent with the postmodern and deconstructivist perspective whereby one's current living situation and the interpretation thereof is the only reality of importance. The social worker is expected to exercise autonomy, creativity, critical thinking, and reconceptualizing abilities, all of which are attributes of the artist. On the face of it this appears appropriate, but it neglects to factor in the reality that most social workers function in bureaucratic organizations with rules, regulations, and proscriptions that preclude the expression of artistic behaviors and judgment. Other than in independent private practice it is highly unlikely that an artful form of social work practice can take place. Most important of all is the fact that social work practice as art does not depend on the application of an articulated base of knowledge and theory. Rather, it depends on skills and behaviors generated internally by the practitioner and applied in a creative fashion to current reality. Social work as art depends on skills acquired from a range of experience and not a knowledge base acquired from a course of study. Artistic practice skills cannot be transmitted from one person to another, which eliminates the need for formal programs of social work education. If indeed social work requires an artful practitioner, it might be necessary to completely rethink the type of preparation and training that would best assist students to acquire that talent. Both beginning and advanced education in the liberal arts appears to be logically more compatible with a postmodern world and artful practice than specific courses in social work of a specialized nature. A postmodern social work education would de-emphasize science in favor of courses in literature, communication arts, history, and the like.

The social work knowledge base as conventionally thought of is also problematic because of its enormous scope, as discussed elsewhere in this book. There are variable levels of human systems, practice technologies, target populations, social problems, and fields of practice for which specific knowledge must be acquired. To master these knowledge areas at a high level of understanding seems on the face of it daunting at best and unreasonable at worst. When this scope and complexity are coupled with the abandonment of the search for theories having multiple applicability, as proposed by postmodernists, the issue becomes further clouded. The vast scope of social work practice interests precludes a concerted emphasis on knowledge development across the variable elements. As a result, social work borrows heavily from the knowledge in other disciplines and professions and then attempts to incorporate it in a coherent fashion. In the translation it becomes watered down and loses its applicability, potency, and relevance. It is an arguable assertion, but there is serious question about the knowledge-building capacity of social work. This assertion gains credibility, as noted previously, when it is recognized that the competence of the editorial boards of professional social work journals, the vehicle for the transmission of new knowledge, is not above challenge (Pardeck, 1992).

IDEOLOGICAL CAPTIVITY

Within the family of health and human service helping professions, social work has experienced and incorporated ideological positions and movements to the greatest extent. Indeed, it may be that social work has become a captive of several ideologies, particularly liberalism, feminism, cultural relativism, postmodernism, and deconstructivism. By "captive," it is meant that some of these ideologies have permeated social work to such an extent that they tend to block out and prevent intellectual dialogue from competing perspectives. These ideologies posit a system of beliefs and assumptions with dual objectives. The first is that they provide an attitudinal, conceptual, and intellectual lens through which to go about examining and understanding the world. The second is a generalized image of what the world should become. An ideologue sees the world within narrow constraints and expends effort to modify the world to fit within them. Ideologies seem to be characterized by the tenacity with which the beliefs are held and by how strongly their adherents attempt to get others to adopt them. It becomes obvious, therefore, that ideologies are a deterrent to dialogue with others who hold dissimilar beliefs. For example, pro-lifers and abortion advocates are unable to communicate meaningfully because of the strength of their oppositional ideological beliefs. The same holds true for social workers who adhere to logical positivism and their postmodern ideological opposites.

In the field of social work there is a long standing ideology that provides a perspective about how social services should be structured. This ideology is liberalism and the compatible offshoots of feminism and postmodernism. It is beyond the scope of this book to fully describe the liberal, feminist, postmodern ideological configurations and comparatively analyze them in relation to conflicting ideologies. Liberalism, feminism, and postmodernism share some similar general beliefs and assumptions. All appear to have a core of perspectives that overlap and view knowledge as relative and traditional science as irrelevant. Each elevates individual freedom over the social contract, disdain for reason in favor of rampant subjectivism and intuition, and the elimination of categories of information across contexts for variations within an infinite number of local knowledge domains. Much to the chagrin of traditional conservatives, morality in a postmodern perspective has no universal standards by which to judge behavior. Indeed, any evaluation of behavior should not be permitted. It is difficult to see how a profession based on postmodernism, such as social work, can survive if it is adrift in a sea of ideological confusion, uncertainty, and chaos. Most important is the fact that it is politically incorrect to adhere to perspectives in opposition to liberalism, feminism, and postmodernism. A belief is held by many, although no empirical studies document it, that conservative social workers are reluctant to submit manuscripts to mainstream journals. They are convinced that social work journal editorial boards have ideological convictions that would preclude acceptance of articles that are critical of liberal and feminist ideas.

THE MYTH OF VALUES

Deeply embedded in the culture of social work is the belief that it possesses an identifiable and unique set of tripartite features of knowledge, skills, and values. These provide the information, the technologies, and, in the last instance, the philosophical grounding and background guidance for practice. The legitimate existence of all three features can be defended more confidently in the first two areas than in the third. There are two problems in understanding what is meant by social work values. The first relates to the essential nature of the conceptualization of values, and the second to their lack of exclusivity to social work.

It is important to distinguish values from related realities that include beliefs, preferences, norms, attitudes, and opinions. The traditional conception of values is that they are inextricably bound to and flow from the larger culture, or population group, and that they function to organize general patterns of behavior within the culture or group. Values are conceptions of the desirable and arise from long-standing shared experiences. Some cultural value orientations are universalistic and arise from transcultural principles and obligations while others are theologically anchored in institutionalized religions. Universalistic, cultural, and theological values are transmitted to and incorporated by persons and serve to inform behavior across a variety of situations and conditions. These values exist outside the person and via socialization are adopted. There are other value orientations of an altogether different order that have an existential and situational anchorage. These values arise out of behavior that occurs in specific situations within a localized context. Rather than existing in the larger culture and being incorporated by the person, values in this conceptualization are created existentially from the freedom to interpret both situation and context. It is an intellectual and conceptual stretch to call these values; nevertheless, they are so designated in contemporary society. More properly they might be considered as beliefs, attitudes, preferences, or opinions.

Values that are frequently identified in social work include acceptance, confidentiality, individualization, self-determination, objectivity, and a nonjudgmental attitude. All of these become problematic within a postmodern model of social work. Postmodernism eschews larger cultural patterns and replaces them with shifting local language communities. It is conceptually difficult to understand how values as defined above are possible within smaller communities that deconstruct and continually recreate themselves. There is a lack of value constancy from one language community to another in that each interprets the value in its own idiosyncratic fashion. The climate of relativism, absolute interpretive freedom, and contextual situationalism in social work are antithetical to the presence of a system of values strongly anchored in the culture at large. What is acceptable in one language community may not be the same in another, or nonjudgmental behavior may vary from context to context. The second problem is that the values proclaimed by social work are not exclusive to it. Certainly, other professions such as psychology, counseling, education, and law espouse a similar value configuration. Indeed, the values listed above likely exist in the larger population to the same degree that they do among social workers. These values do not, therefore, constitute a unique feature of social work.

PROFESSIONAL ETHNOCENTRICITY

The fundamental orientation, perspective, and approaches within the tradition of American social work are so entrenched that they can only be described as ethnocentric in that they are viewed as superior to social work in other countries and cultures. When course outlines in social work education programs are reviewed, rarely does one find a text or a required reading from a journal published outside the United States. Social work practitioners and social work educators routinely visit other countries to provide consultation, program design, and development. Yet it is a rare occasion when social workers from other countries are invited to the United States in the hope that they can contribute to our version of practice. Social workers in other countries have approached the disparities in social provisions, the problems of oppressed peoples, and social injustice issues along different lines than in the United States. In this country, even though there are dozens of specialized fields in which social workers practice, most of them follow a form of practice that is either direct service (clinical) or the administration and management of social service agencies. Neither of these practice approaches is particularly relevant to the improvement or elimination of poverty, the creation of opportunities for disenfranchised groups, or the elimination of systemic social injustice. These are all major elements in the overall purpose and mission of professional social work, yet the overwhelming majority of practitioners employ methods with little relevance to them. Sadly, in the person-in-the-environment niche, the focus is on the adaptation of the person to the environment rather than changing the environment itself.

The human service approach most appropriate to deal with systemic problems and issues is called social development. Social development is the modality most evident in countries outside the United States, particularly those classified as third world, developing, or underdeveloped. As a practice approach it is somewhat abstract since it includes a philosophy about helping and a conceptualization for change as well as a set of objectives. Nevertheless, it differs from clinical and social administration approaches. It attempts to link both social and economic sectors of the environment to make them more responsive to human needs, aspirations, and problems in a developmental rather than remedial and residualist fashion. Many distinguished social work educators and theoreticians have articulated the social development approach and its utility (see for example, Billups, 1990; Estes, 1990; Karger, 1994; Midgley, 1990; Beverly and Sherraden, 1997). But even though the literature about social development is increasing, it does not appear that it has had a significant impact on the world of daily practice or on social welfare policies. The only social work journals that regularly publish social development material are *International Social Work* and *Social Development Issues* and both of these have a rather low number of subscribers. Although social development holds great potential for moving social work in the United States toward an intersectoral, structural, and institutional change orientation, its adoption on a wide scale is unlikely. The presence of the clinical focus and the orientation toward maintenance of existing bureaucracies are so firmly entrenched that a new modality has little chance of making an impact. In spite of the criticisms that have been presented about the postmodern approach, it does possess features compatible with social development. These include the restoration of social power to the local level, the removal and subsequent replacement of institutions antithetical to local needs, and emphasis on the subjective interpretation of reality in place of external metanarratives imposed from outside. A goal for mature social work in the United States would be the elevation of social development approaches to the same level as clinical and social administration. Apparently, market forces do not indicate a need for social workers within a social development mode. A review of social work job announcements for a two-month period did not include one advertisement for a social agency seeking a social development practitioner.

POSTMODERNISM AND OTHER "ISMs"

In an attempt to logically connect the mission of social work with the educational establishment and the actions of practitioners, the profession has reached out and embraced a number of contemporary perspectives. These perspectives purport to provide ways to better understand and deal with what is perceived as the chaos, uncertainty, and ongoing rate of change characteristic of the late twentieth century. Chief among these is the perspective called postmodernism, which shares characteristics compatible with social constructionism, feminism, cultural relativism, and existentialism. Each of these latter perspectives is a radical departure from traditional theoretical and scientific modes of viewing and studying reality and attempts to understand the person in the environment. Each of these perspectives in its own fashion challenges the methods, premises, and legitimacy of logical positivism and traditional modes of science.

Even though the several "isms" differ in important ways, a central core of beliefs and assumptions conceptually binds them together (Meinert, 1998). Chief among these is that objective reality does not exist; that it is a specious exercise to create universal categories of experience; that the generalizability of knowledge is not possible; that metanarratives or grand theories need to be deconstructed and destroyed; and that traditional empirical science has tended to deny "subjugated knowledges" (Hartman, 1992) that exist among the marginalized of society. Also running through these assertions is the belief that reason and logic must be replaced by locally anchored intuition and subjectivity. In this view, therefore, it is impossible to develop universal knowledge and generalizable statements since valid knowledge can only be generated by participants in local language communities. To believe otherwise is to encourage external control and power by observers outside the local group.

The proponents of postmodernism for social work and social work education (Pozatek, 1994; Sands and Nuccio, 1992; Weick, 1993) base their convictions on a series of fuzzy assertions about social reality. A new conceptual and philosophical paradigm is proposed for the profession which, when examined closely, has no agreed-upon elements or structure. There appear to be as many definitions of postmodernism as there are postmodernists. The entire postmodern movement lacks a clear explanation of what it means. It is not a theory, nor does it contain a set of systematic and organized conceptual propositions that can be tested. That is perhaps consistent with one of the tenets of the perspective, which asserts that reality is socially constructed and that there are as many realities as there are definers of it. It consists, therefore, of a constantly changing medley of interpretations, none of which can be applied to other situations and conditions.

Social workers who were trained prior to the appearance of the postmodern influence are taken to task for exerting the power of their knowledge over clients. Their actions are also called into question when they apply the generalizations learned from other situations and contexts to the reality at hand. Many who are both postmodernists and feminists believe, wrongly in the view of the authors, that reality is interpreted in a fundamentally different manner by women and men. Albeit there are shades of difference in the interpretive process, it is a big leap to believe that women lack the same attributes of reason and objectivity to the same extent as possessed by men. Also, no compelling evidence supports the idea that men lack the intuition and subjective abilities of women. But it is logical from the postmodernism feminist perspective to connect the attributes of women, intuition and subjectivity, with the denigration of traditional science based on reason, logic, and objectivity. Little attention has been paid to the counterargument advanced by a leading female epistemologist and equity feminist that women have capacities equal to men in performing traditional science (Haack, 1992). It is disrespectful of women to argue that they are less proficient in mathematics, abstract reasoning, objectivity, and rational thinking than are men.

SOCIAL WORK AND SOCIAL POLICY

The traditional dual focus in social work on assisting persons and families to improve their social functioning and on having an impact on the larger environment is well documented. The second focus involves activities on several fronts, one of which is the development of social policies that support social justice and human betterment. The accreditation standards and curriculum policies for social work education are very explicit about the need for students to develop competencies in the social policy area. At the undergraduate level the expectation is the acquisition of analytic skills, and at the graduate level not only analytic skills but the ability to influence policy formulation and actually change it (CSWE, 1992a, 1992b). Upon completion of training, practitioners have the responsibility to work at both developing policies that enhance the mission and objectives of social work and changing existing policies that impede these objectives. The social policy process itself has four main phases involving formulation, legislation, implementation, and evaluation (Pardeck and Meinert, 1994). Policy activities take place at various levels including national, state, community, and organizational. The focus for social work at the several levels pertains to relevant fields of human need such as mental health, child welfare, income maintenance, developmental disabilities, and the like. A fair assessment of the record of social workers in the social policy process at the several levels across the various fields is that its impact has been minimal and is undistinguished at best.

Four main reasons support the above conclusion. First, as noted elsewhere in this book, the boundaries of social work are extraordinarily expansive, particularly in terms of numerous fields of practice that take place at all levels of human systems with variable technologies. This results in policy interests in all the fields of practice with minimal effectiveness in issues that cut across them all. Second, social policies that have the greatest impact are ones directed at national and state levels (macro). Most social work effort takes place at the organizational or community levels. Third, there is clear evidence that most social workers have a desire to follow clinical careers. This is not to assert that they have no interest in policy within the larger context, but that most of their focus is on what takes place locally. Finally, over the past few decades an ideologically oriented political philosophy rooted in conservatism has permeated the citizenry, and it has strongly influenced the formation of national and state social policies. Most social workers are overwhelmingly liberal in ideology and are outside the mainstream of policy development. Last, of the four phases of the policy process—formulation, legislation, implementation, and evaluation—social workers are essentially out of the loop with the first two and minimally involved with the last two. In some fashion social workers are more reactors to social policy than creators of it. There are, of course, some notable exceptions to the above analysis. Persons such as Harry Hopkins, Whitney Young Jr., Jane Addams, and Wilber Cohen had enormous impact on national social policy. It would be difficult, however, to develop a list of dozens of social workers who now operate and had an impact such as they did.

STATUS OF SOCIAL WORK EDUCATION

As described and concluded elsewhere in this book, social work education has been a higher education success story. The number of programs, students majoring in social work, and faculty instructing them continue to increase in number without any sign of letting up. As the official sanctioning body for social work, the CSWE has developed an elaborate structural mechanism and a process to accredit programs that is accepted and appears to work well. But when an exploration takes place that looks below the surface and examines the underlying curricular logic, some areas of concern appear. Three concerns of major import in social work education relate to program need, curricular positioning, and validity of the knowledge base.

During the preliminary stages of the accreditation process, institutions must clearly document that there is a community need for the program. This documentation must go beyond the simple judgment that a need exists and include actual data from community leaders, agencies, and potential students. The documentation also must demonstrate that graduates of the program will have sufficient employment opportunities. Following the granting of initial accreditation, at subsequent accreditation reviews this standard is never again raised. The result is the questionable need for many programs and a geographic maldistribution of programs. At the undergraduate level the five states with the lowest combined population (Wyoming, Alaska, Vermont, North Dakota and Delaware) have ten programs for 2,871,717 citizens. The five states with the highest population (California, Florida, New York, Pennsylvania, and Texas) have ninety-nine programs for 89,556,555 citizens. For the low-population states this is one program for every 287,171 citizens, and for the high-population states this is one program for every 904,611 citizens. There is a disproportionate number of small liberal arts colleges in low-density states. They serve small geographic catchment areas with a smaller prevalence of social problems, yet they have proportionately more BSW programs. Many of these BSW programs have only two faculty and a small number of majors. The programs are situated in very small liberal arts colleges and two faculty teach all the social work courses, which provides students very little instructional variety. On the other hand, there are BSW programs located in huge universities with numerous faculty and an extremely large number of available cognate courses. It is difficult to view the small programs as equivalent to the large ones, yet they are seen that way by the CSWE. It would seem prudent for the CSWE to attempt to have some influence over the geographic distribution of programs on the basis of regional need. It has never conducted a study to ascertain where the need for BSWs and MSWs is most critical or where there is a surfeit of programs.

Another concern is the focus and placement of educational content between the baccalaureate and master's levels. At the BSW level it is broader and more extensive in scope, while at the MSW level it is narrower and more specialized. BSW students are expected to master content embracing many levels of human systems and population groups in multiple fields of practice employing a variety of helping techniques. At the MSW level the content is specialized. Compelling arguments can be made that this should be reversed.

Two concerns are present about the social work knowledge base. The first relates to the extent to which it is confirmed and valid. The second is whether knowledge production in social work is deficient and whether that which is produced is used in practice. Howard and Lambert (1996) point out that the low production of relevant empirically based and practice-oriented research has hindered the acceptance of social work by the public. The antiempirical stance of many practitioners in their view could lead to the denigration of social work as a major profession. At the graduate level only a very small percentage of students are in doctoral programs. Most of these programs do not emphasize training in research to the same extent as doctoral programs in other disciplines. After social workers receive doctorates, their publication rate is very low. In a study by Baker and Wilson (1992), only half published after graduation. All of these conditions do not bode well for the social work knowledge base. It also appears that social work journal editorial boards may not be competent to perform that function, which may be related to the quality of the published articles and the low impact of the journals themselves (Howard and Lambert, 1996).

SUMMING UP THE CHALLENGES

The challenges facing social work as it moves into the new century may not represent the beliefs and opinions of the majority of those in the profession. The authors are convinced, however, that the questions raised in this chapter are legitimate ones after having examined all aspects of the profession. They are equally convinced that efforts must be undertaken to restructure social work if it is to remain a viable partner in the system of major social and human service professions. A beginning in the analysis and restructuring is to assess the degree to which social work possesses the first-order integral attributes of professionalism and admit that it falls short on some. Questions have been raised about the negative consequences of the postmodern movement in social work, which is increasing while at the same time the presence of science-based practice is diminishing. The knowledge base of the profession is of debatable legitimacy. Presently there are over sixty social work journals and their number increases annually. They span many fields and, while they steadily increase in number, the quality and competence of their editorial boards is suspect.

The central direction for social work is now generated from an entrenched liberal, postmodern, and increasingly feminist ideological perspective. This tripartite configuration seals itself off from other perspectives and deprives the field of conceptual and theoretical input that could expand its intellectual diversity. Indeed, social work has become a champion of diversity in all areas other than the intellectual. This rigidity also prevents social work from becoming a major factor in the development of social policies for a new century characterized by malleable and shifting political agendas. All of these observations indicate a professional system that has closed itself off somewhat to new thinking from outside itself. As such it is now in an entropic stage, which must be altered in order to survive and flourish in the coming century.

Chapter 2

Crisis in Social Work Theory: Can a New Spirit for Social Work Be Constructed Out of the Shattered Grand Narratives of the Past?

After examining reasons for the collapse of the grand narratives of social work as a profession, the authors apply a model suggested by Kitchin (1998) to review what the major streams of theory in the social sciences have to offer social work today. Next the authors propose a foundation for a new spirit or zeitgeist for social work that might arise from the ashes of the old narratives.

The history of the grand narratives in social work is intimately intertwined with the industrial revolution (Wilensky and Lebeaux, 1965) and its consequences on one hand (poverty and inequality, segregation and discrimination), and with theories derived from academic psychology and sociology (Gomory, 1997). These theories were meant to account for conditions brought on by massive social change (Dodgshon, 1998), and were in turn used to justify palliatives for social work as a profession (Brennan, 1973). During the most recent postindustrial period, the decline of the Communist bloc and the ascendance of the profit sector have dramatically altered the structural foundation of social work once again (Abramovitz, 1986; Stoesz, 1997; Bryner, 1998; Meinert, 1998), greatly diminishing the influence of the public sphere while witnessing the continuing commodification of social work practice (Karger and Stoesz, 1998). The public sector has been co-opted by the profit sector, as demonstrated in the managed health care movement in the United States. A critical consequence of this phenomenon is that traditional grand narratives which guided social work as a profession have been shattered into dozens of smaller pieces (Kuhn, 1970). According to Tolson (1988):

The amount of information available to social workers in the form of models of practice and research findings has increased tremendously in the past few decades. The information is difficult to employ because there are no unifying conceptual structures. (p. 19)

What specifically accounts for the decline of the grand narratives in social work as a profession and why have the auspices for public policy been undermined? After examining four factors that may account for the downfall, the authors use Kitchin's model for social science theory to speculate on the components of a new spirit for the profession.

DECLINE OF GRAND NARRATIVES

The first factor that has helped to destroy the grand narratives in social work involves the demise of the nationalistic traditions and cultures in capitalist countries, because of what Agger (1995) called "fast capitalism." Fast capitalism has eradicated the common cultural centerpiece for mutual aid (Karger and Stoesz, 1998), so important for justifying help to those victimized by the industrial revolution. But how does fast capitalism destroy grand narratives that traditionally support the activities of social work as a profession?

It is ordinarily through socialization that each generation is provided with the foundation to build mutual aid for the next (Trattner, 1974). But in societies undergoing fast capitalism, children are likely to have little common understanding of the role of public welfare and the common good. For example, according to Ritzer (1992), children in the United States today are intimately familiar with electronically engineered histories attached to assorted market-generated cartoon and fantasy characters (e.g., Barbie dolls and Luke Skywalker), but because such stories have nothing to do with a common heritage, they are not likely to stimulate interest in political and cultural grandeur, nor the mutual aid commitments suggested therein. The snowstorms of pixel images that radiate outward from electronic industries drive frenetically toward the creation of a generation of children raised to behave as hyperconsumers responsive to hypermarkets (Baudrillard, 1988).

Specialists tell us that postindustrial economies throughout the world now require massive amounts of electronic titillation generated by the private sector in order to move products through various market centers (Poster, 1995). Perhaps this is the reason why those who design suburban shopping malls find it necessary to create perpetual springtime inside, substituting plastic participation and cyber reality for the natural landscapes of forests and streams belonging to the previous generation. Today, middle-class suburban children do not leave home prepared to meet public landscapes familiar to previous generations, who were loaded down with fishing poles and sack lunches. Rather, children depart home today carrying portable circuitry and plastic credit prepared to engage in busy consumerism in the marketplace.

Participatory narratives, which traditionally tended to bind members together under the umbrella of one huge cultural superego (Poster, 1995), have been replaced by microstories that could well have been created by graphics specialists in the Netherlands. But instead of binding members together in one cultural experience, these market stories by their very nature appeal narrowly to the primal urges of the id. Portable electronic paraphernalia assure that these micromessages are received without passing through the filters traditionally available in the family or peer group. Instead, such consumerist stories are broadcast to each isolated individual about his or her own suggested behavior in the marketplace, maintaining a secret relationship between advertiser and consumer that eats away at communal values.

Without the basic myths and legends supporting a commonly held philosophy, the communality of mutual aid so important in an industrialized society has faded away. Like a locally owned, family-operated store bought out to make room for a suburban megamall, the recognizable traditional participatory culture of the United States has likewise been bought out (Baudrillard, 1988). Filling the void are borderless worldwide corporate superstructures generating market stories about everyone in general and yet no one in particular, while presenting computer-generated advertising landscapes somewhere and yet nowhere (Lefebvre, 1991). Such market-driven forces have transfigured the public welfare landscape and, in combination with the other three factors discussed here, have effectively undercut the foundation for social work's grand narratives.

Second, massive demographic dislocations in the third world have had profound consequences upon international markets in food, clothing, and shelter, leading in these early stages to the development of worldwide supernetworks of producers and distributors (Ohmae, 1995). These master economic systems perforce require transportation systems and communication channels that jump easily over governmental boundaries of individual nation-states, as witnessed in the push for North American trade agreements and the newly emerging European Union. Eventually, population pressures require the production of goods and services of such magnitude that the rationale for locality-specific regional governance is circumvented. Social work as a profession has lost its primary public auspices and nationalistic value orientation. As Ohmae (1995) predicted, modern nation-states are no longer adequate for dealing with the threats and opportunities of the global economy.

In the short run, this means that once-vibrant communities in the United States have bifurcated into barren landscapes for the poor and limited-access homogenized villages for everyone else. Drucker (1993) sees this phase as a form of tribalism. That is, for the short run, distinct groups which formed the traditional clientele for social work will continue to define and identify themselves in terms of linguistic, religious, and cultural communities which they can comprehend and embrace.

Even now, social work plays no role in the microurban areas containing corporate schools, artificial rain forests inside shopping malls, and company-owned cemeteries that are under construction in new communities attached to theme parks, with access limited to select demographic groups via deed restrictions and other socioeconomically oriented discriminations. According to Gottdiener (1985, p. 15), "The present is witness to the progressive marginalization and spatial confinement of those social groups least able to play an active role in the political economy."

The third factor that has assured the end of grand narratives in social work involves radical changes in our orientation to physical space and land made possible by a set of bold new computerized hypertechnologies. These new computer-generated physiopsycho-social systems will obsolete the relationship between clinicians and the world around them. In addition, instead of commuting to nearby business, factory, or leisure-time locales, cyberwork will become available entirely at home. The social worker and client as both producer and consumer will thus be physically and socially isolated from each other. The typical clinician or client will only be tied vertically, via modem and other electromagnetic satellite linkages, to worldwide systems which will span and eventually trivialize local, regional, and national public boundaries and the human service delivery systems contained therein. There will be no need for local and eventually regional and national cultural and social systems that provide the auspices for social work practice.

A vast array of new technologies will obsolete current local competitive skills as obstacles in daily work rounds will be overcome in totally electronic computerized personal territories. Just as innovations in petroleum refinement beginning in the 1960s in the United States obsoleted blue-collar skills in heavy industry (Manchester, 1974), so too will we find our distinctly American know-how everywhere made available to everyone. No society will corner the market in any one skill area, as even the slightest microskill will be performed by prosthetic devices available to everyone by satellite linkage.

Innovative and undreamed of cyber environments, that go way beyond simple computer terminals of today, will produce electronically engineered idiolectic cyberspaces that will physically and psychologically encompass the individual. Brahm and Driscoll (1995) warn that these prosthetic territories, involving the boundary between humans and machines, portend a ". . . new terrain of political and cultural struggle [in] . . . hybrid spaces of theory-practice . . . between the 'cybernetic' and 'organism' " (p. 3).

The fourth and final factor that has splintered the grand narratives of social work includes a wide range of genetic and chemical solutions emerging as researchers complete the search for material that may soon describe the entire human genetic code. Even the definition of life as an "extended phenotype" is given new meaning in keeping with a genetic orientation to the gene pool as having a distributed existence. According to Dawkins (1986, p. 171): "The long-lived gene as an evolutionary unit is not any particular physical structure but the textual archival information copied down through the generations." In the global corporation-dominated borderless world envisaged here, the private sector will control all types of genetic productivity, including the commodification of reproduction.

The historical significance of breakthroughs in genetics and chemistry as sciences is similar to the situation in classical physics 100 years ago. In the mid-1890s many trained in traditional physics felt that there were no new discoveries to be made, that the knowledge base for science had reached its limits (Lindley, 1993). A few scientists warned of major cracks in the foundations of then-modern physics, however, which we now know began to crumble with the publication of Einstein's paper on relativity in 1905. The implications of the relativity theory shocked the societal value base at that time and quantum physics soon brought X rays, radar, television, atomic energy, and much of the modern electronic computer world (Lindley, 1993).

Today, those who prophesy about the emerging evolution in genetics (Gibbs, 1995; Dawkins, 1995; among others), have similarly warned us that it is but a shockingly small step from the Human Genome Project to the complete restructuring of human DNA. Although residual chains of specific prodromal (potentially disease causing) genetic material may escape such engineering, findings suggest that a large number of physical and psychological problems will soon be amenable to genetic amelioration (Whelan and Black, 1982). According to Lapham (1996, p. 1) ". . . the risk to all of us is biological determinism, and we need to resist this."

Even now we read of weekly breakthroughs in genetic testing and recombinant DNA solutions for diseases and germ transmission. It is not difficult to envisage a genetically engineered, comparatively disease-free future in the next fifty years. Other currently perplexing problems will find similar solutions, though there may be shocks to societal value bases as well. In the years ahead, population pressures and uncertainties in current conception control policy and practice may lead to the eventual genetic manipulation of reproduction in men. The male genetic code might be rewritten to limit male fertility to restricted periods of productivity, thus all but eliminating unwanted pregnancies, need for termination of pregnancy, and the like.

A future dominated by genetic preventionism affords little or no opportunity for intervention by the rest of us. A recent analysis by Dawkins (1995) captures the logic of DNA determinism:

Humans have a rather endearing tendency to assume that "welfare" means group welfare, that "good" means the good of society, the well-being of the species or even of the ecosystem . . . [but in] . . . a universe of electrons and selfish genes, blind physical forces and genetic replication, some people are going to get hurt. . . . DNA neither knows nor cares. DNA just is. And we dance to its music. (p. 85)

Accompanying the DNA revolution are dramatic advances in the highly profitable chemical industry. Breakthroughs in quantum physics (Lindley, 1993), and the development of quasicrystals (Greenwood, 1992), foreshadow an emerging field of affect-chemistry in which medication triumphs over problems in living. Countless new combinations of molecules will permit novel chemical solutions so that many human conditions not amenable to genetic manipulation will be subjected to hypermedications, thus altering what we understand to be the feeling component. According to Gibbs (1995, p. 105), "Already some well-respected behavioral scientists are advocating a medical approach to crime control based on screening, diagnostic prediction and [chemical] treatment."

But what does this situation portend about the grand narratives in social work? In an effort to help construct a replacement framework which we call the new spirit, we apply a model suggested by Kitchin (1998), which provides a foundation for generating key questions from the narratives.

UNDERSTANDING GRAND NARRATIVES IN SOCIAL WORK

There have been a number of characterizations of the theoretical and philosophical foundations of social work as a profession. Excellent discussions of various theoretical approaches are available in Stretch (1967), Forder (1976), Krill (1976), Germain and Gitterman (1980), Barker and Hardiker (1981), Hearn (1982), Whittington and Holland (1985), Turner (1986), Banton (1987), Dore (1990), Greene and Ephross (1991), Howe (1995), Lischman (1991), Mullaly (1997), and Payne (1997).

Kitchin (1998) maintains that there are six fundamental perspectives for viewing discussions of innovations in social sciences. Each perspective captures a slightly different aspect of how theories can be viewed in social work and the kinds of questions each perspective might raise. Here we have extended Kitchin's basic model to include a fuller account of his sixth perspective, which he identifies as feminism. We extend this perspective to include all participants or potential participants who are not currently empowered, and we broaden the category from feminism to the polyvocal narrative.

Utopist/Futurist Narratives

According to Kitchin (1998), utopist and futurist narratives seek to forecast how innovation will affect future conditions on a societal scale. Such forecasters claim societies are moving en masse to some new and novel stage and that many vexing problems today will be subject to radically new scientific solutions in the future (Reisch and Gambrill, 1997). In the social work literature, Kreuger (1997) and Stoesz (1997) both foresaw an end of the social work profession after the collapse of public auspices due to the decline of the nation-state during the postindustrial era. They include advances in technotherapies and hypertechnological prosthetic territories and a decline in the grand narratives of the profession as indications of the end of the profession as a whole. To the futurists and utopists, the narratives are powerless to stop the inevitable force brought on by massive structural changes. Utopists and futurists claim there is little hope of directing changes coming upon the profession and that it would be well served to learn to accept and adapt to massive structural change.

Determinist Narratives

The determinists argue that social, cultural, political, and economic aspects of our lives both as professionals and in the private sector are individually determined at the micro level by narratives. Narratives, themselves not caused by social factors and essentially inevitable, are the dominant shapers of society (its social structure) and culture (the way we think and act). Narratives are seen as independent, active, and determining (Chernus, 1995), and the profession is seen as identity dependent, passive, and reactive. According to Karger and Stoesz (1998), the determinist approach in social work is evidenced by the privatization movement, which encourages social work managers to define success solely in terms of efficiency criteria, but not to choose to reject what may be, in the long run, problematic choices on the effectiveness side.

Constructivist Narratives

The social constructivists argue that metanarratives must be seen strongly as a social construct and that they cannot be separated from their application, but rather are intimately entwined with each other and with nature (Habermas, 1987). Individuals are free, from this perspective, to interpret narratives in any of a number of alternative ways (Reamer, 1993; Booth, 1994).

From a constructivist approach, traditional positivism is seen as unable to examine its own assumptions about objectivity apart from the manipulation of numbers (Payne, 1997). Qualitative researchers express a constructivist view in rejecting predefined research categories, insisting on inductive (theory free?) investigations, and viewing the world from within the context of the participant in a phenomenological sense (Heineman, 1981).

Political Economy Narratives

Those who advocate the perspective of political economy suggest that the relationship between narratives, society, and social work as a profession is bound within capitalist modes of production and the associated political, economic, and social relations that underlie capitalism and its extension to social work, privatization (Banton, 1987). The private sector is the dominant shaper of social policy and practice, and narratives help to reproduce social relations of the private sector so that the balance of power tends to remain the same (Epstein, 1995). Narratives are rarely neutral (Karger, 1986), but are developed in the interest of industrial and corporate profits. From this perspective, a narrative is little more than the latest ideology of the capitalist state, ever perfecting and thrusting the profit motive into the lifeworld (Mullaly, 1997). From this view nothing can ever be transcended.

From this perspective, a number of purely profit-oriented systems are dominating the landscape of ideas worldwide while specialized language is ensuring that access is restricted to a relatively privileged few (Wise, 1997). Energy that was formerly available for helping and healing is now being spent on practices which amount to a kind of object fetishism. That is, we may be at a period in the history of social work when we are sacrificing sound practice in the field for busy consumerism in the office (Kreuger, 1997).

Postmodernist Narratives

Postmodernists criticize all that the past 100 years of modernity has engendered, including industrialization, urbanization, and the nation-state (Chambon and Irving, 1994). This perspective (Murphy and Pardeck, 1998) sees the profession moving to a culture that denies depth and history, a profession in which alternatives are always mixed and blended (Howe, 1994), and a culture of pastiche, superficiality, and "depthlessness" prevail (Harvey, 1989). Economic and political systems have been evolving with a global movement away from the local (Conner, 1989), accompanied by a vast restructuring (Epstein, 1990). We are living in times of fragmentation (Imre, 1984), decentering, disorientation, and disenchantment (Pardeck, Murphy, and Chung, 1994), as we wander about in the postindustrial phase. Theorists focus upon meanings of identity (Norris, 1993), the body (Foucault, 1990), and community and place (Berman, 1982; Lefebvre, 1991). According to Kitchin (1998), these concepts are bound up and affected by the social production of time and space and the blurring of boundaries between reality and virtuality, nature and culture.

Polyvocal Narratives

The feminist perspective recommended by Kitchin (1998) suggests that narratives are dominated by, and reflect, the position of men; specifically, white, wealthy, Western men. Here, we extend Kitchin's feminist perspective to include any persons not currently empowered and fully participating in the discussion and shaping of narratives (see, for example, Davis, 1985; Collins, 1986; Saulnier, 1995; Longres, 1997). The narrative space created by the profit sector, like earthspace, is not developing as a viable location for those not already intimately involved due to their underpositioning on account of lack of power.

We want to extend this final perspective to include any set of persons not currently empowered and able to participate in the universal transcendental community.

The utopist/futurist narratives in our view are overdetermined and contrary to the whole perspective of the new spirit. On the plus side they suggest, however, that we need to improve our efforts to gather much better data to assess how practitioners, clients, and those in training adapt to different forms of temporal and spatial distance, how they relate to the emerging aspects of electronic communication over distance, and how they adapt to individual differences in reception of ideas.

From a determinist narrative, continued dialogue, discourse, and debate through traditional or specialized national forums in social work on the proper role and consequences of metanarratives and their impacts on the natural environment are encouraged. The physical, social, and interrelational helping environments should serve as the active consideration and operative criterion for judging the costs and benefits associated with each narrative as it reflects the international workplace.

From the constructivist narratives, professional boards and oversight committees associated with standards, licensing, and codes of ethics should demand a focus on achieving more humane outcomes. This in turn suggests that wholesale application of specific market interventions and commoditylike treatment in social work requires thorough review.

From the political economy narratives, social work as a profession needs to adopt a policy statement that demands free public access to the entire electronic assemblage of hypermodern technology and free public terminals available and accessible to all without regard to position in various national and international marketplaces. If we are indeed on the way to becoming "terminal citizens," then we must demand access for all.

From the postmodernist narratives, as Wise (1997) suggests, alternative narrative structures are needed that do not isolate people from their socioeconomic and political environs which shape what should be our professional agendas in such areas as poverty, racism, and sexism. According to Baudrillard (1988), everyday life is increasingly conjured by market images and object-oriented discourse that substitute for hard-and-fast reality in areas of traditional social work concern such as poverty, racism, and sexism. In this regard language no longer positions itself in a passive representational relationship to reality such that words clearly and cleanly describe an existing world. Instead, language, including writing, has become a muddy, ambiguous medium that necessarily defers clear understanding indefinitely, thus obfuscating the role of structure in determining life chances.

Finally, from the polyvocal narratives, alternative structures are perhaps more difficult to specify simply because there are so many voices to be heard. Theorists such as Appadurai (1990) argue that a global culture promised by polyvocal narratives produces not democracy, but cosmopolitanism, which has unclear implications for social work, especially in the third world. On the other hand, Habermas (1987) claims that multiculturalism and diversity issues evoked and registered via polyvocal metanarratives amount to "market-administered conversations," which are incapable of getting beyond the code to even begin to discuss a truly universal transcendental community. According to Agger (1998):

> Multicultural theory valorizes polyvocal perspectivity and denies logocentric, Eurocentric, androcentric privileging. Perspectival knowledge, articulated in the small narratives of everyday experience and vernacular, is at once partial (nontotalizing) and inherently valid, given the intimate relationship between what Habermas called people's knowledge and interests. (p. 177)

PROLEGOMENA FOR A NEW SPIRIT FOR SOCIAL WORK

An effort to rethink the problem of the shattered grand narratives in social work during this postmodern period engages a number of complex issues. Particularly difficult is the struggle to outline areas of concern without being seen to authorize interests when no particular frame of reference or set of experiences can be called upon for justification. Nonetheless, let us see what might be offered up using as a foundation the concerns raised earlier in this chapter, in what is called the search for a new spirit for social work.

First, in conceptualizing a new spirit for social work we must resist premature closure of inquiry and investigation by rigidly conceptualizing closed, bounded categories of thought for our theories and theoretical constructions, operational definitions, or for the sweeping grand explanations of history or the micronarratives of various polyvocal subject positions. We need rather the capacity to combine creatively what may have been portrayed in the past as oppositional categories, such as varieties of race, gender, or caste. We must question what Soja (1989) called the "totalizing deep logics" that incapacitate our creativity. We need to allow ourselves to find novel combinations to take shape ". . . unburdened by the biases of the past but guided by the testing ground of praxis" (Soja, 1989, p. 73). Finally, we oppose "otherness," the conceptual marginalization and subordination of various groups of people and their practices. According to Agger (1998), many social science narratives ignore "other" voices or relegate them to a role outside their zone of attention.

Second, a new spirit for social work must be built upon a deeper exploration of the critical silences in the professions regarding domination by the profit sector. This is particularly true in regard to the wholesale disregard many in the profession have for mixing practice effectiveness with profit taking. We need to attempt to elaborate a new spirit (or new spirits) for social work as a profession that reverses the imposing tapestry of the past (Soja, 1989), exposing the intellectual history of the profession and its relation to the profit sector.

Instead, our efforts must be grounded in the political and theoretical demands of contemporary international movements and able to encompass all theoretical and vocal forms, from what Soja (1989, p. 74) calls the "grand strategies of global geopolitics to the 'little tactics of habitat.'" Our reconstituted new spirit or zeitgeist must be attuned to the emancipatory struggles of all those who are peripheralized and marginalized, such as exploited workers, tyrannized peoples, and dominated gender.

Third, we must recognize the importance of the body in local as well as grand narratives. Every narrative, whether it be a story of actualization or the narrative of an individual's growth and development, should be credited for confirming the narratives of emancipation of humanity or the achievement of the transcendental community.

A critical element in our new spirit for social work is the human body and its relation to what is ordinarily called nature. Concerns about aging, death, genetic engineering, organ transplants, growth hormones, physical trauma, diet, and a host of other concerns demand attention in the new narratives. According to Murphy (1997):

> What is missing in all these theories is the continuing importance of the dynamic processes of nature that regulate human bodies and the interaction of such processes with social action. The body has been perceived as a receptor of meanings, whereas it should be seen as a generator of meanings. (p. 44)

According to Murphy, the distinct approaches to narratives about the human body include the mannequin theory, which describes the body as an inert object that is embellished, decorated, and presented according to particular values. This is a social construction approach to the human body and only examines how discourse produces the body. The next narrative, according to Murphy, sees the human body as a living organism that is experiencing the processes of nature, such as growth, decay, disease, and eventually death—the living organism theory. The third narrative, which is socioecological, is more inclusive and holistic, according to Murphy. This narrative properly positions content about human beings in a broader environmental context including concerns about pollution and conservation. It situates the human body:

> as a living organism in its context of other living organisms and of the dynamic, interdependent processes of nature, including other ecosystems such as the air, water, minerals, and soil, with radiation from the sun and the gravitational pull of the earth. (p. 47)

Fourth, the destabilizing power of various professional interest groups needs to be recognized, as they have already reinforced the splintering of the profession into pockets of specialities, each with its incompatible language game. None of these language games should have superior claim any longer to external principles of justice or authority. In this situation, the specialties, according to Conner (1989), seem to have adopted a goal of "no longer truth but performativity." No longer do they seek what kinds of research will lead to emancipation or transcendence, but what kind of research will work best, where "working best" means producing more research of the same type, thus promoting the opportunity for even more research.

Universities and institutions of higher learning have not in these circumstances been so concerned with transmitting knowledge in itself, but have been tied ever more narrowly to the principle of performativity, so that questions no longer concern matters of truth, but rather performance and cost (Conner, 1989).

Fifth, we must explore ways to become "negative heroes" by virtue of our capacities to carry out intellectual guerrilla war inside the system, by making destabilizing moves in the language games of increasingly market-generated authority (Poster, 1995).

Sixth, we need to support the building of new public spaces, which refers to any regions freely accessible to all, whereas "private places" refers to soundproof regions where only members or invitees gather— the traditional concern for public order beginning only at the point where a private gathering begins to obtrude upon the neighbors (Goffman, 1963). From the perspective of the new spirit, new public space should support the principle that the public life of a community is dialogically available to a free community of inquirers. According to Fischer and Karger (1997):

> A reconceptualized social work practice must be framed in a vision of public life, social change, and a progressive common good that unites oppressed classes and aggrieved groups. (p. 180)

There should be opportunities for free speech acts in Habermas' sense (1987). There should be a capacity to recognize and experience social relations as historical accomplishments that can be transformed. According to Agger (1991):

> . . . in trying to restore the public sphere [we] must not renounce its [the public sphere's] theoreticity. The world is complex and must be theorized complexly. The postmodern aversion to theory is symptomatic of a stupid age. This is not to say that theorists should constitute a new vanguard but only to note that the attack on mandarinism and elitism must be tempered by the recognition that we have a very long way to go before we can use a genuinely critical public discourse unproblematically. (p. 15)

In this regard, we need to develop strategies that help to overcome what Baudrillard (1988) called the market-structured bogus interaction in social work, which creates audience muteness. That is, activities that seem like public behavior to those involved but are not:

> A mass medium broadcasts to its audience, while never [actually] allowing that audience to respond to it and, indeed, confirming the audience's muteness by simulating audience response, via phone-ins, viewer's polls, focus groups. Against this synthesized communication is an ideal of free, immediate exchange, in which the hierarchical split between the transmitter and the receiver is transmuted into a mutual responsiveness and discursive responsibility in spontaneous dialogue. (p. 53)

Seventh, our final concern involves the recent movement in social work toward many of the new hypertechnologies that have emerged in the last few years. Evidence from the field (Tenner, 1997; Thurow, 1998) shows that while more administrative reports are being generated containing fewer spelling errors, more and more paper is being consumed but spelling is not improving among social work students. We are sacrificing the depth of social work's strong suit, interpersonal insight, for the breadth of the wide open but shallow spaces of electronic networks. Such spaces lend themselves to the pursuit of complicated electronic solutions to trivial problems (Kreuger, 1999). We are substituting hypertechnological rigor for practice relevance.

SUMMARY

The history of the grand narratives in social work parallels the industrial revolution and applies theories derived from academic psychology and sociology. During the recent postindustrial period, the structural foundation of social work has been altered by fast capitalism, diminishing the influence of the public sphere while the private sector has ascended to a dominant role. After examining reasons for the collapse of the grand narratives of social work as a profession, the authors applied a model suggested by Kitchin (1998) to review what the major streams of theory in the social sciences offer today. Finally proposed was a foundation for a new spirit or zeitgeist for social work which might arise from the ashes of the old narratives.

Chapter 3

The Disjuncture of Science and Social Work

Over four decades ago, Greenwood (1957) published an important article that attempted to analyze the professional status of social work. He argued that it is critical that a field possess the following attributes to achieve full professional status:

1. A systematic body of theory
2. Professional authority
3. Community sanction
4. A regulative code of ethics
5. A professional culture

Greenwood (1957) concluded the following about the professional status of social work:

> When we hold up social work against the model of the professions presented above, it does not take long to decide whether to classify it within the professional or nonprofessional occupations. Social work is already a profession; it has too many points of congruence with the model to be classifiable otherwise. (p. 44)

Greenwood also noted that the power and privileges of a profession are extended to members through the acquisition of education designed to prepare individuals for professional life.

Even though Greenwood presents a convincing argument about the professional status of social work, a number of writers have challenged his position (Pardeck, Chung, and Murphy, 1997). Collins (1975), a sociologist, offers convincing evidence that social work has not met the core criteria to be classified as a profession and that it remains a semiprofession. He suggests that this lack of professional status is largely due to the fact that social work continues to lack a systematic theoretical base that grounds practitioners in a common approach to practice. Collins suggests that the field of social work lacks a clear theoretical base due to the tension between social work and science, with science being referred to as a traditional epistemology grounded in an objective approach for discovering truth and developing knowledge.

UNEASY RELATIONSHIPS BETWEEN SOCIAL WORK AND SCIENCE

Mace (1997) argues that a number of reasons help to explain the tension between social work and science. One most often suggested is that practitioners typically are frustrated by the lack of relevance of research findings to direct practice. According to Mace, research offers little help with the day-to-day decisions made when working with clients. Mace (1997, p. 150) concludes that "we are stymied by our inability to make predictions even for our client's simplest behaviors."

Mace suggests that social work research follows a reductionistic model grounded in the physical sciences. In essence, it attempts to reduce phenomena to a limited number of independent variables for explaining client behavior. Clearly this model has been very successful in the physical sciences; however, according to Mace, it has limited utility for social work practice.

Mace (1997) argues that human beings are far more complex than phenomena found in the world of the physical sciences. Individuals cannot be easily broken down into component parts that allow for scientific investigation. Human beings are extremely complex entities and the environments that they interact with add to this complexity.

Furthermore, according to Mace, the social sciences have produced no widely accepted constructs about human behavior. Science has not provided a sound theory to explain the nature of human beings and why they behave as they do. Furthermore, much of the theory guiding the social sciences is largely untested and thus offers little to enhance social work practice (Mace, 1997).

Keeping these issues in mind, the dominant theory guiding social work practice is the ecological systems perspective (Kilpatrick and Holland, 1995), a theory that clearly suffers from many of the criticisms presented by Mace (1997) concerning the uneasy relationship between social work and science. The ecological perspective offers a comprehensive model for explaining human behavior in the context of the social and ecological environment. The following summarizes the major underpinnings of the ecological systems perspective.

THE ECOLOGICAL WORLDVIEW

The core assumptions that guide the ecological perspective are presented below. As can be seen in this list, the ecological perspective is clearly a holistic approach that includes the individual, family, organizational setting, community, and the larger social ecology. The following assumptions create the grounding for the ecological perspective:

1. Transactions are understood as being contingent upon reciprocal exchange guiding behavior.
2. Life stress can be seen as positive or negative within the person-environment relationship.
3. Coping is seen as part of the problem-solving process and the management of dysfunctional behavior.
4. Habitat is the social setting in which individuals reside.
5. Niche is the result of the individual's accommodation to his or her environment.
6. Relatedness in one's environment supports attachments within the social ecology.

Systems Theory

Systems theory is an important theoretical grounding of the ecological perspective. Systems theory supposedly helps the practitioner to understand how the client system is influenced by and influences the larger social ecology. It is a theoretical approach that moves away from a reductionistic view of human behavior by stressing wholeness as the key to understanding individual social functioning. Component assumptions of systems theory are as follows:

1. Wholeness suggests that change in one part of a system causes changes throughout a system.

2. Feedback regulates a system by inputs.
3. Equifinality suggests there is more than one way to get to a final state.
4. Circular causality is not grounded in cause-and-effect interaction. Systems theory views linear thinking as being extremely limited as a guide to understanding human behavior.

Practice Focus

The ecological perspective, with its heavy emphasis on systems theory, provides the following guidelines for social work practice:

1. The interactions between individual and family are critical for understanding social functioning.
2. Practice roles are conducted in a person-in-the-environment context.
3. An important aspect of practice is to focus on the life cycle and transitions within this cycle.
4. The focus is on strengths, not deficits, of clients.
5. Assessment occurs at multiple levels including micro, mezzo, and macro.

Limitations of the Ecological Approach

As Mace (1997) suggests, the ecological perspective is largely untested. It appears to be more of an ideology than a sound scientific theory. Given this position, the following summarizes the limitations of the ecological perspective:

1. The individual and family system must adapt to the environment; this kind of adaptation may be viewed as oppressive.
2. Homeostasis is a goal. Change thus may be seen as negative.
3. Systems subordinate individuals, families, creativity, and autonomy.
4. Little or no scientific validation has been offered supporting the ecological perspective.

The ecological systems perspective is comprehensive, offering practice guidelines for intervention at multiple levels. In fact, the Council on Social Work Education accreditation guidelines mandate that the ecological systems perspective must be covered in social work programs (Commission on Accreditation, 1994). The problem, however, with this mandate is that the systems perspective has not been validated by methods using rigorous scientific methodologies. Even though the ecological systems perspective "feels right" and offers a grounding for combining both policy and practice, it lacks validation through the traditional epistemology of objectivism. Given this situation, and as suggested earlier, the field of social work may well be driven by a perspective that appears to be grounded more in ideology than science. The history of social work has a long tradition of practitioners relying more on ideology than science as their basis for practice (Thyer, 1997). If the field of social work continues to reject the core assumptions upon which objectivism is based, it is unlikely under these conditions that a sound social scientific theory will emerge as a guide to practice.

OBJECTIVISM VERSUS CONSTRUCTIVISM: SOCIAL WORK'S UNEASY RELATIONSHIPS

Fisher (1991), a constructivist, claims that the field of social work should abandon the traditional constructs of the social sciences in favor of a constructivist epistemology. Borrowing from Fisher's work, it will be suggested that the field of social work has been grounded heavily in a constructivist epistemology since its founding. In a certain sense, social work as a field has been postmodern since its inception. What has emerged from these conditions is a weak knowledge and theoretical base that seems to be interpreted and reinterpreted by each new generation of social workers.

Objectivism versus Constructivism

Objectivists and constructivists (Fisher, 1991) offer uniquely different worldviews for knowing and understanding human behavior. Objectivism has been the dominant epistemology in Western culture. Constructivism has also been present in Western thinking; however, it has been clearly overshadowed by objectivism (Fisher, 1991). Table 3.1, based on Fisher's work, provides the basic tenets for each approach to understanding the world and ultimately human behavior.

As can be observed in Table 3.1, the objectivist epistemologies present a much different view of the social world than the constructivist epistemologies. The objectivist view suggests that reality is independent of the person, whereas the constructivist approach argues that reality is created by each individual. Truth is relative according to the constructivist approach, whereas the objectivist worldview concludes that truth is absolute. Knowledge development, in the objectivist approach, results from the categorizing of concepts; the constructivist orientation views knowledge as fluid. The constructivist understands science as a process unique to the observer; the objectivist views science as the core methodology of discovery.

Even though the profession of social work publicly endorses the objectivist approach to discovery, the heavy reliance on "practice wisdom" as the dominant strategy for guiding practice suggests that the

TABLE 3.1. Objectivist versus Constructivist Epistemologies

Objectivist	Constructivist
1. Reality exists independent of the person.	1. Reality is constructed by the person.
2. Absolute truth can be uncovered.	2. Truth is relative to time and place.
3. Knowledge consists of verifiable facts.	3. Knowledge is a social construct.
4. Meaning resides externally to symbols.	4. Meaning is a result of social interaction.
5. Knowledge results from categorizing concepts.	5. Knowing is an ongoing process of interpretation of events.
6. Science is the core method for discovering truth.	6. Science is an interpretive process unique to each observer.
7. Causality can be discovered.	7. Causality is a complex process involving numerous elements.
8. Individual behavior is determinate and can be understood.	8. Individual behavior is indeterminate.

profession appears to be heavily influenced by the constructivist approach. Given this tradition, the field of social work continues to define and redefine itself with each new fad that emerges in the popular literature. The result is a weak knowledge base that has limited grounding in sound theory. Under these conditions, theory development is often chaotic; each collective of social workers has their own unique idiosyncrasies in which they ground their practice worldviews. The lack of knowledge boundaries within the practice of social work means the field will continue to have problems finding a niche among the helping professions. The remainder of this chapter will focus on the key issues that have resulted from the field's disjuncture from science. Science is the pinnacle of objectivism. A sound knowledge base for social work practice will only emerge from a greater emphasis on science in the field of social work.

RESEARCH TRAINING AND EDUCATION

By rejecting an objectivist epistemology, the field of social work places itself outside the mainstream of academic life. This has resulted in questionable academic standards within the field of social work. The lack of commitment to science also ensures that the profession has

limited status and influence within the academic community. In turn, disciplines that are grounded in science, such as psychology, political science, and sociology, are well established within the university setting.

Midgley (1999) notes that social work has a checkered history in academic institutions and particularly in major research institutions. Social work is typically criticized by the humanities and sciences because it does not emphasize scholarship and rigor. Midgley goes on to note that among professional programs, law and medicine are often seen as the more rigorous programs within the university community; social work most often is viewed as the least. This status within academia has extremely negative consequences for the profession. As long as the profession continues to reject the importance of science as the core modality for discovering knowledge and rests its theoretical base on ideology and "practice wisdom," the status of social work will continue to be low.

A major factor that has contributed to this lack of status within the university community is the emphasis on the MSW degree over the doctorate of social work. As has been clearly noted within the official Council on Social Work Education accreditation guidelines, the MSW is considered the terminal degree (Commission on Accreditation, 1994). In fact, it is often confusing to university officials when they discover that there is a doctoral degree in social work, yet the MSW is considered the terminal degree by the profession and the Council on Social Work Education.

This extremely unusual circumstance can be attributed to the small number of doctoral graduates produced in social work each year. Graduates have been few since the inception of doctorate programs of social work. In 1964-1965, only 39 people received a doctorate in social work; by 1989-1990, the figure rose to 247 degrees received. From 1985 to 1990, an annual mean of 9,282 MSW degrees was reported (U.S. Department of Education, 1993).

Other disciplines produce much greater numbers of doctorate-level graduates. For example, in 1990-1991, 5,272 doctoral degrees in engineering were granted, 2,238 doctorates in chemistry, and approximately 252 doctorates of social work. Graduate schools of social work are not producing enough doctorate-level social workers. This appears to have resulted in the profession's limited commitment to research and virtually no knowledge development based on traditional scientific approaches (U.S. Department of Education, 1993).

Spaulding (1991) reported that approximately 45 percent of faculty members in graduate-level social work programs do not have doctorate-level training. Obviously, it is easy for faculty lacking doctoral education to miss the importance of science as the basis of knowledge development. Spaulding also reported that only a small number of recently graduated doctorate faculty in social work were exposed to the latest research methodologies. Green, Hutchinson, and Sar (1992) found nearly 50 percent of doctoral-level graduates in social work had a tendency not to publish in professional journals after receiving their degrees. This lack of commitment to scholarship only contributes to the low status of social work within academia.

Jenson, Fraser, and Lewis (1991) report that many social work programs lack solid research foundations. For example, one-fifth of the programs require one or no statistics courses. Approximately half required two research classes. This kind of standard appears to have resulted in a large number of doctorate-level social work graduates having poor preparation in the area of research. This lack of commitment to research at the doctoral level is even more pronounced at the MSW level. Jenson, Fraser, and Lewis (1991) conclude:

> Research training in social work is a prisoner of an out-dated paradigm. Focused largely on casework training at the MSW level, this paradigm insures that doctoral students will enter doctoral programs with weak research methods and statistics backgrounds. In the absence of greater vertical integration of research content, social work appears likely to remain a profession dependent, in large part, on other disciplines for knowledge generation. The fundamental structure of social work education must be reconsidered if the profession is to make a serious effort to generate its own research knowledge. (p. 37)

There appears to be virtually no continuity between the BSW, MSW, and doctorate levels in required research courses (Fraser, Lewis, and Norman, 1990). This means agencies employing social work graduates have no idea of the research capabilities of a recent graduate from a school of social work regardless of the degree earned. A meaningful commitment must be made to ensure that social work graduates have an appreciation for the importance of science in knowledge development. Graduates also need to know how to use research methodologies to produce knowledge.

Obviously the lack of commitment to science within the field of social work has resulted in deficiencies in scholarly productivity. As mentioned previously, nearly half of doctorate-level graduates have never published an article in a professional or academic journal. Abbott (1985) also noted that the modal number of articles, books, and book chapters was zero for social work faculty. Given these findings, what criteria are used to grant tenure and to promote social work faculty since large numbers of faculty never publish? If tenure and promotion are being granted based on nontraditional criteria, it becomes clear why social work has limited prestige within the university community.

The fact that scholarly productivity among social work faculty is so limited clearly does not promote the viability of social work within the larger society. It is extremely important that this situation be changed to ensure the survival of social work in the twenty-first century.

THE SOCIAL WORK LITERATURE

Refereed journals play an important role in the development of new knowledge within academic disciplines. The editorial boards of journals are critical in determining what articles will be published for public dissemination. Since the 1970s a number of studies have been conducted exploring the scholarly productivity of social work editorial boards. As would be suspected, the editorial boards of most social work journals fall short. This circumstance raises serious concerns about the quality of the literature that is published in the field's journals.

In the 1970s, Lindsey (1976, 1977) found that social work editorial boards lack distinction and achievement in scholarly productivity. Lindsey measured productivity on the basis of the number of articles that members of editorial boards had published and how often they were cited by others in the literature. Recent research by Pardeck (1992a, b) replicated much of Lindsey's research conducted two decades earlier. Pardeck found that social work editorial boards continued to lack scholarly achievement.

A recent study by Pardeck and Meinert (1999) even suggested that the profession may be less than honest about the low quality of its editorial boards. In their research, they found that one of the leading journals in the field, *Social Work,* claimed that all members of its editorial board were experts in their areas of specialization with strong records of publication. Furthermore, tenure committees gave high marks to those publishing in *Social Work.* Pardeck and Meinert found, however, that 50 percent of the editorial board of *Social Work* from 1990 to 1995 had not published an article and the other 50 percent were cited three times or less by others. The consulting editors for *Social Work* had similar records of publication. Nineteen percent had not published during the time period studied; nearly 25 percent were cited three times or less from 1990 to 1995. These findings are consistent with the profession's lack of commitment to scholarly productivity. They are more telling, however, because the policy of *Social Work* is to appoint only individuals with strong publication records—not following a stated policy clearly weakens the credibility of one of the most important journals in the field.

As might be suspected, those who explore the research productivity of social work editorial boards do so at their own risk. Pardeck (1992a, p. 487) concluded that research on editorial boards is sparse because "critical examination of social work editorial boards could be aversive to editors and perhaps result in deleterious consequences for the critic." An example of negative consequences include events surrounding Epstein's (1990) research on editorial boards. Epstein reported that his research resulted in the National Committee on Inquiry of the National Association of Social Workers nearly banishing him from the field. Epstein found in his research that social work manuscript reviewers were frequently inaccurate, incoherent, and lacked an understanding of basic research methodology. Epstein (1992) concluded that research findings by Pardeck (1992a, b) are simply another example of the poor intellectual climate of the field of social work:

> Social workers on editorial boards are drawn out of the undistinguished base of social work academics. Large numbers of tenured professors, even in prominent schools of social work, have never published anything. For others, productivity halted after being awarded tenure. Many appointments to social work faculties have little to do with teaching, scholarly, or intellectual competence. They seem to have a lot to do with the traditional varieties of corruption (nepotism, cronyism, trading favors, and the fecundity of incompetent selection committees in replicating themselves) and their New Age variants (compensatory appointments on the basis of gender, race, sexual preference, and ethnicity and political correctness). An undergraduate degree in social work today does not certify literacy. A graduate degree does not certify competence. An appointment to a social work faculty does not certify merit. (p. 527)

Lindsey (1999) more recently confirmed Epstein's concerns. Lindsey reported that not only are nonscientific and idiosyncratic standards often used by social work editorial boards, but are also employed by schools of social work when they select faculty for chaired professorships. He found that a number of major research universities that have endowed professorships allow faculty to be appointed to these positions based on criteria other than scholarly merit. For example, one person was appointed to an endowed chair at a major university without one significant publication to that person's credit. Another prominent university with an endowed chair in social work appointed a person to the chair who had virtually never been cited in the literature by others. In contrast, at the same university, but in the sociology department, a distinguished scholar was appointed to an endowed chair who had been cited in the literature extensively by others. Lindsey's findings offer another example of why the profession of social work lacks standing in the academic community.

The poor quality of social work editorial boards has the result that other disciplines pay limited attention to the social work literature. Cheung (1990) reported that social work journals cited psychiatry, sociology, and family studies journals 4.7, 5.4, and 2.3 times more often between 1981 and 1985 than they were in turn cited by journals in these respective fields. Epstein (1992) concluded that the impact of social work journals is astoundingly low. For example, the *Social Science Citation Index* in 1989 reported that *Social Work* and *Social Services Review* had impact ratings of .73 and .45. These two journals are arguably the most prestigious in the field. These scores are far below the impact ratings of major journals in psychology, political science, and sociology.

Finally, Fraser et al. (1991) found that the quality of research published in social work journals is very poor. They investigated fifteen social work journals between 1985 and 1988 and discovered few articles that used systematic data collection technologies. The use of any experimental design was almost nonexistent in the social work literature. Most findings relied on rudimentary descriptive or univariate research approaches. The poor quality of research in social work journals reflects the inadequacies in the research education of graduate schools of social work and in the evaluation process of articles. It is important to graduate more doctoral-level social workers and to place greater emphasis on science in all aspects of the social work curriculum. Until this is done, the quality of published research in social work journals will continue to suffer. The status of social work within the university community will only increase if the profession begins to adhere to the canons of science as the basis for knowledge development.

SCIENCE-DRIVEN PRACTICE

Kirk (1990) and Schilling (1990) found that many social workers do not rely on empirical findings as a basis for their practice. This discovery is partially attributed to the poor research training social workers often receive at the graduate level. A strategy that might assist professional social workers to rely more heavily on empirical findings as the foundation for their practice might be to publish a clinical guide that outlines interventions that have been found to work effectively (Pardeck, 1991). A number of fields, including medicine, have used this kind of technology.

A number of years ago, the single-subject design showed great promise (Brian, 1990); however, the enthusiasm for this technology quickly subsided. Brian observed the following about empirically based technologies:

> That the empirical practice movement has had little impact on the profession at large other than social work education is not surprising for two reasons: one reason is that advocates of empirically based practice have made little effort to reach the profession at large, beyond publications and sessions at a few conferences. Second, many researchers have greater access to social work education than to organized social work. If we researchers think it is important to have a greater impact on the profession at large, other than the long-range impact through students, then we will need to consider what it would take to accomplish that goal. (p. 6)

Gingerich (1990) concluded that social work practice is largely based on "practice wisdom," not empirically tested practice. Like Kirk (1990), Gingerich feels that there are limited resources for and commitment to developing and testing social work interventions. Given this situation, it is unlikely in the near future that the field of social work will use empirically based research to guide practice. Until there is a greater commitment to science, the status of the field will remain low among the helping professions and within the larger academic community.

SUMMARY AND CONCLUSION

The field of social work has limited commitment to science as its source for knowledge development. Even though the Council on Social Work Education accreditation guidelines identify research as an important curriculum content area (Commission on Accreditation, 1994), the research reports that this curriculum area at all degree levels, bachelor's through doctorate, is weak.

A sound theory base for practice has not emerged because there are simply not enough doctorate-level graduates in the field. Furthermore, doctorate programs often do not provide the research rigor needed to test the hypotheses underpinning theory development. The field's treatment of the MSW as the terminal degree means that demand for doctorate-level-educated social workers has not emerged. The MSW curriculum simply does not enhance an appreciation for research nor the importance of research in testing and building theory. Given this situation, the field will continue to struggle because of its weak theoretical base—which means limited professional standing among other helping professions and disciplines.

The uneasy relationship between social work and science must end. Even though Mace (1997) suggests that science has little to offer social work practitioners, he is simply wrong. In fact, Thyer (1997) would argue that such a view may be unethical because it suggests Mace has not explored the numerous available effective technologies that work. These technologies have been thoroughly tested through the scientific method. Science has much to offer social work practice, and it must play a central role in the knowledge development of the field.

Given the lack of commitment to scientific rigor in the field of social work, it makes perfect sense that individuals without strong qualifications are appointed to social work editorial boards. It is also evident why individuals would be appointed to endowed professorships without a single publication or citation of their work. Science helps to ensure standards that include criticism of new ideas and knowledge. When ideology is the underpinning of a knowledge base and scientific rigor is suspect, which appears to be the case in social work, the contructivists and postmodernists can push the agendas in the field.

In a recent article by Duncan Lindsey (1999) focusing on ensuring standards within the field of social work, he found empirical evidence documenting the lack of commitment to research as well as academic standards within schools of social work. The following quote from Lindsey's work succinctly captures the current state of affairs in the field of social work:

> The few cases I have illustrated here are being repeated many times over through the profession. Although I believe they are due largely to a kind of hidebound, inflexible habit or traditionalism that has failed to recognize the imperatives facing the profession, mutterings of cronyism and favoritism are now being heard from many corners My concern is that many talented and gifted researchers have grown disillusioned, with some so disillusioned they are ready to abandon the entire field as unsalvageable. Certainly, until we are resolute in upholding research standards, we will be failing our clients and in danger of failing as a profession as well. (1999, p. 119)

Chapter 4

Hypertechnology in Social Work

The postindustrial period of social work practice has transformed much of the more mundane everyday practice wisdom into scientific knowledge (Karger, 1983); created new agency environments while casting off old ones (Gandy and Tepperman, 1990); speeded up the whole tempo of social work practice without necessarily increasing effectiveness (Kreuger, 1997); initiated new forms of organizational power and struggle for control among varying age, gender, ethnic, and class lines (Gottdiener, 1985); caused upheavals in skill levels and training needs (Stretch and Kreuger, 1992); generated numerous ethical concerns in treatment (Reamer, 1986; Cwikel and Cnaan, 1991); and severed colleagues and clients from their traditional habitats (Ritzer, 1992); hurling them from their known worlds and into new technologically dominated lives (Poster, 1990).

In recent years, social work has been inundated by sophisticated and often costly hypermodern technology (see for example, Iacono and Kling, 1996; Conklin and Osterndorf, 1995). Following Wise (1997), we use hypermodern technology (or hypertechnology) to refer to "not just one piece of equipment, but the entire interconnected assemblage of technologies . . . which share a formal resonance or common episteme" (Wise, 1997, p. xvi). It is our position that the carefree early frontier days of hypertechnology are over. It is no longer possible to discuss one application or piece of equipment apart from the economic and political hypertechnological sphere, which forms a much larger assemblage. Commercial interests (Thurow, 1998), now direct and govern the hypertechnology landscape in every arena, including social work education.

This chapter was co-authored with John J. Stretch.

We want to consider a range of possible consequences that this commercial technological assemblage may be having for social work. As Wise (1997) points out, purely market-based profit motives are dominating the technological assemblage worldwide, which is restricting access to a relatively privileged few. There are reports that the manufacture of hypertechnology is exploiting workers and their families in the third world, and that the environment is being despoiled during production.

Discussions available in the social work literature on hypertechnologies ordinarily report on one aspect or application of hypertechnology at a time. For example, there have been reviews of the role of technology in social work in general (see Phillips and Berman, 1997, on simulation (Wodarski and Kelly, 1987), virtual realities (Brooks, 1997), cellular and telecommunications devices, microcomputers (LaMendola, 1987; Seabury and Maple, 1993; Monnickendam and Eaglestein, 1993; Patterson and Yaffe, 1994; Howard, 1995; among others), Internet linkages (Giffords, 1998), videodisc media (Lynett, 1985), and related applications (Reamer, 1986, Born, 1987; Cnaan and Parsloe, 1989; Caputo, 1991; Saleebey, 1991; Schopler, Abell, and Galinsky, 1998; Siegel et al., 1998; Memmott and Brennan, 1998).

Over the past several years, practitioners and those who educate for practice have been increasingly pressured to adopt hypertechnology, but they have not been given supportive data regarding the positive outcomes technology promises. It is almost as if decision makers have been motivated by a fear that their agencies or departments will be left out (Perelman, 1992). The train is leaving the station and everyone wants on board, but no one has any idea where it is headed.

The authors contend, moreover, that we may not have kept pace (except see Schopler, Abell, and Galinsky, 1998) with the implications of these pedagogical innovations either in terms of the organizational changes they are causing (in the ways we teach and therefore how students learn) or the impacts they are likely to have on practice (Blakely, 1994; Conklin and Osterndorf, 1995). In addition, a host of mechanical and technical troubles have been identified by Tenner (1997), which educators need to anticipate as technology begins to bite back. The authors summarize a number of issues concerning hypermodern technology in social work education and offer suggestions for educational policy and practice.

WHY DO WE HAVE HYPERMODERN TECHNOLOGY IN SOCIAL WORK?

So much new hypertechnology has been generated that we now find ourselves rushing to justify expenditures on technology in most every academic and practice setting. We do so not because we are convinced that these ventures will enhance client self-determination or improve access to scarce resources, but because we are caught up in a cybermachine ideology. The authors argue that we may be slowly destroying key foundations of traditional social work in the process.

Social work has recently begun adopting a number of new methods of producing and distributing information and knowledge, loosely organized around the themes of openness (Paul, 1990), distance technologies (Siegel et al., 1998; Thyer, Polk, and Gaudin, 1997; Warriner-Burke, 1990), offices and campuses without walls (Brindley, 1989), and video and computer-assisted communication (Carey, 1991).

Traditionally, social work agencies and academic institutions were characterized by closed environments (Hawkins, 1991), typified by communication contained solely within bounded physical space utilizing locally available resources. These traditions paralleled the social and economic organization of the larger surrounding community. According to Connick (1997), local educational institutions were organized in accordance with their industrial heritage, which included centralized campuses (similar to factories), proximity of students and faculty (organized as workers and managers), and adherence to a strict academic schedule (production cycle).

But the postindustrial period has transformed the nearby organizational environment from an industrial to an information-based setting. At the same time in the education arena, the end of the World War II baby boom witnessed a dramatic decline in the number of younger learners entering college, forcing institutions to compete for increasingly older adult learners.

But the recent wedding of distance-spanning innovations (Perelman, 1992), information technology (Jones, Kirkup, and Kirwood, 1993), and telecommunications (Johnstone, 1991) into powerful new structures has served as a catalyst for a paradigm shift that is well under way, according to Connick (1997):

The digital age will allow us to move images of every sort far more efficiently and cost-effectively than we can move people. We will be able to connect students or clients and others to the experience they need, in real time or asynchronously, regardless of whether it is by voice, video, or data. (p. 11)

OFFICES WITHOUT WALLS
AND DISTANCE-SPANNING INNOVATIONS

Paul (1990) contends that the major variable in various models of open campuses and distance-spanning innovations is the extent to which the individual, rather than the institution or the profession, gains control over the educational process. According to Paul such control includes: (1) how something is learned (organization of materials, various media, and teaching methods), (2) where it is learned (at home, in a regional center, on campus, or anywhere in between), (3) when it is learned (start dates, self- or institutionally paced), and (4) how it is assessed.

But the use of one-way and synchronous television and satellite communication has created a host of potential pitfalls for the social work practitioner and educator (Biner, 1993). Unlike face-to-face interaction in conventional classrooms, where both professor and student share in the creation and execution of the present moment, electronic technology has instead restricted the knowledge of clients or students to available photographic images, and likewise, clients and students experience flattened and truncated two-dimensional views of their professors or clinicians. According to Dede (1991) faculty must decide whether to adopt a more attractive "telepresence," which might take the form of a pleasing character from television such as Mr. Rogers.

Traditional classroom instruction is considerably different from the ordinary everyday telecommunications that students observe at home. As Zigerell (1991) points out, "Students watching a program in geology or psychology this morning . . . may very well have viewed exciting episodes of *L.A. Law* or *Mission Impossible* the evening before." Further, in the 1990s, exposure to an average of forty-five hours per week of electronic media assured that the typical student witnessed 17,000 murders and over 16,000 acts of sexual intercourse by the time he or she reached age eighteen (Kubey and Csikszentmihalyi, 1990). According to Dede (1991) distance technologies do not use traditional methods for communicating with students because they rely on the visual in contrast to auditory environments.

In a national survey of distance education in schools of social work, Siegel and colleagues (1998) report the following problems: the limiting of instructional materials soley because of the demands of technology-assisted instruction; problems in developing and maintaining faculty preparation; scheduling and network synchronization demands that may disrupt the ebb and flow of learning; insufficient institutional support; and decreases in the amount of personal contact among faculty and students.

Thyer, Polk, and Gaudin (1997) reported, "Our preliminary comparison of student assessment of live instruction versus distance learning found a significant difference in favor of live instruction . . . our data suggest caution prior to its widespread adoption" (p. 365). The 1986 Annenberg/CPB report indicated considerable dispute in deciding on the value of distance education. Such instruction offers "no educational advantages over traditional media for the same population of students" (Kling, 1996).

COMPUTERS, THE INTERNET, AND RELATED HYPERTECHNOLOGY

Human service agencies and schools of social work are reporting a never-ending push to acquire and upgrade several of the newer microtechnologies including computer-assisted instruction, Internet courses, and the like (McWilliam and Taylor, 1996). How is the energy expended on new technology impacting other nontechnological aspects of social work education? Is the equipment worth the cost, especially when faculty and students seem to be spending more and more of their time interacting with objects and less time in one another's presence? Sassone (1992), for example, reports that many highly trained professionals are spending more of their energy engaged in what amounts to secretarial and clerical projects. According to Iacono and Kling (1996):

When real gains in productivity are measured, people often find new tasks that exploit the gains. Consequently, extra working capacity does not necessarily translate into cost reduction or even improved overall effectiveness. (pp. 312-313)

Birkerts (1996) maintains that while computer networks may be seductive places to work, play, and communicate, they remove professionals even further from the ebb and flow of the natural helping network found outside the classroom:

> There is a tremendous difference between communication in the instrumental sense and communion in the affective, soul-oriented sense. We are, as a culture, as a species, becoming shallower . . . we are adapting ourselves to the ersatz security of vast lateral connectedness . . . faith in the web. (p. 82)

O'Reilly (1980) found a negative correlation between the amount of information people had to do their jobs and the quality of their actual performance. According to Sproull and Kiesler (1996), "Economists point out that people often overinvest in information, they acquire more information or more costly information than they need to do their work" (p. 471). Birkerts (1996) claims that while textual messages can be sent across a computer net in a few milliseconds, conversations and other meaningful life experiences, which have been the staple of social work interventive healing relationships (see, for example, Stretch, 1967), require much longer periods of time to unfold.

The authors have observed that new forms of hypertechnology have been instrumental in the establishment of new organizational systems containing new power relations and new ideologies for educators and practitioners alike. In schools of social work we see this expressed as competition among administration, staff, faculty, and students for access to equipment as a scarce resource. And in the larger practice community, according to Gottdiener (1985) local political cultures are dying out partially due to the increase in the number of individuals who are isolated by technology from the community that surrounds them.

Increasingly elaborate forms of microtechnologies available to ever-larger numbers of human service professionals, students, and faculty over progressively larger territories has eroded the centrality of face-to-face conduct, helping to create what Fisher (1995) called "communities without propinquity."

WHAT IS WRONG WITH HYPERTECHNOLOGY IN SOCIAL WORK?

The cybermachine ideology that accompanies hypertechnology has helped to destroy social work's traditional grand narratives and the deep structural socioeconomic agendas we share as a profession. We have witnessed increasingly the trivialization of social work knowledge (Epstein, 1995), the McDonaldization of human services delivery (Kreuger, 1997), and recently the ascendance of cyborg logic. A cyborg is, according to McWilliam and Taylor (1996):

> Effectively, a human-technology fusion, a fantastic body that is not collapsible onto anatomy, gender, or sexuality but is a body that is all and everything. The cyborg processes, in the words of Sofia (1995, 153), "a polymorphously perverse fantasy body that can possess combinations of organs not found in nature." (pp. 168-169)

Specific problems with hypertechnology in social work practice and education for practice are outlined in the following sections.

Lack of Theoretical or Value Orientation

Hypertechnology lacks a theoretical or value orientation to guide development and set or adjust program priorities. Academicians and practitioners alike have been caught with their theoretical pants down in accommodating imperatives coming from hypertechnology that disrupt traditional practice forms (Pickering, 1995). We can find no published conceptual framework for dealing with hypertechnology and no sense of paradigm shift to help assimilate it.

Research in social work is ill-equipped to deal with hypertechnology issues because of an epistemology that focuses on the sociopsychologistic turn at the expense of any other. Add to this an administrative superstructure that is caught up in its own circular logic, and we end up endorsing the technologically driven move to disembodied campuses and agencies without walls, for example, without any empirical support whatsoever. According to McWilliam and Taylor (1996):

> For the highly successful lecturer or thesis supervisor, the fact that she/he is no longer standing and delivering to students

who are materially present may be experienced as disembodiment, as the loss of means by which she/he introduces students into a discipline. When teleconferencing students complain, as they do when telephone lines are unclear, that the teacher is "breaking up" or "fading," the teacher who never "cracks up" in terms of lecturing or tutoring performance, may experience a profound sense of loss of control over the work in which she/he was once so practiced. (p. 167)

Reduction of Availability with Increase in Distance

Hypertechnology in social work is slowly eating away at presence availability (Giddens, 1984) while at the same time increasing time-space distance. Students and clients alike are increasingly being isolated from centrally located spatially packed resources, including diminished access to practitioners and faculty. Consequently, social integration and the mutual monitoring of behavior can no longer occur through face-to-face communications in intimate locales such as the workplace, in the household, or in conversation. According to Gottdiener (1985):

> Contemporary transformations in the space-time matrix of social organization have fundamentally altered the conditions of local community life. The spatial segregation of social groups has liberated the vast majority of the population from responsibility for the less advantaged . . . [involving] the progressive marginalization and spatial confinement of those social groups least able to play an active role in the political economy. (p. 269)

We can only guess at the long-term consequences of these conditions, but we speculate with Warf (1991) that the microelectronics revolution has created increasingly sterile hypermobile human-serving industries which escape traditional stewardship constraints in seeking out private sector profits.

Hypertechnology Scene #1

It is very quiet in the telecommunications room where you are waiting for someone on the other end to get a microphone working so that you can actually hear the demonstration lecture which is supposed to be broadcast between 2:00 and 2:30 p.m. In the hypertechnoworld everything now begins "on the hour" because of the temporal synchronicity required by international satellite hookups.

Anticommunity Narratives

The narrative (story) of hypertechnology is largely anticommunity. We are concerned that hypertechnology achieves anticommunity by requiring forms of communication (modems, e-mail) which ultimately destroy communal participation, creating a dialectical tension that threatens the realization of the distant dream of community (Fisher, 1995). New forms of hypertechnology have been instrumental in the establishment of new production systems containing new power relations and new ideologies for educators and practitioners alike.

Hypertechnology Scene #2

You are standing too near when suddenly, like an angry bear stuck on the wrong side of a lake, the fax machine begins to emit irritatingly loud, variably pitched, machine-generated telephone screechings, bouncing around the walls of the mail room. Without getting too close you scan the unhelpful icons on the input area of the equipment and decide you are powerless to quiet the effrontery of this office beast. Of course, you've heard this before, so now you are hoping for a shrill notification that things are going to quiet down soon when the machine finally connects to its partner on the other side of the lake (end of the line).

Hypertechnology suggests a negative heuristic, which in turn sacrifices the lived experience of clients, practitioners, teachers, and students. We agree with Marcuse (1964) that technology's danger lies in its totalizing nature, for to control machinery is to exercise political power. The rationalization required of social work practice and educational settings through hypertechnology has created political, economic, and technical elites who eventually come to control consciousness itself.

Hypertechnology Scene #3

> You are typing a letter using your office microcomputer when suddenly the keyboard freezes up . . . the cursor is stuck on the far left side of the page and nothing you do will get it moving again. The only thing left to do is to quit working on the letter, hope some of it got saved, and start over. Next time, save your work more often.

It seems to us that as a profession we have come to believe that goals can presumably only be achieved by convincing all interested parties to define happiness solely in terms of the technological choices, but not to choose to reject wasteful consumption to begin with (Ferre, 1995):

> The root of the new technological repression lies in consciousness itself, the elimination of the chance for the Reason of Plato to function in its gadfly role. When everything present is affirmed, when everyone is happy, then imagination itself is crippled in its power to take account of the absent, to long for what is not. Marcuse realizes that the surly refusal to "go along" with the rational society must appear neurotic . . . (p. 71)

Loss of Freedom

Hypertechnology causes profound losses of personal freedom, obfuscating the fact that few are any better off. Although supposedly involving only contentless, passive educational or supportive service delivery systems, hypertechnology actually represents the height of materialism in the ascendancy of the tool to replace the individual and the stories we tell. Hypertechnology tends to hide the question of how it got to where it is, who really benefits, and what its implications are. According to Gottdiener (1985), hypertechnology has created a society where:

> Local community life loses the street and public areas of communion to the [techno]-privacy of the home. Neighbors be-

come increasingly estranged through a lack of common experiences, despite the superficial appearance of civility between them, as the personalized network replaces the localized community of the past, with its once dense social relations. The new areas of communion are encapsulated within the social worlds engineered by the logic of [techno-]consumption—the malls, shopping centers, singles bars, amusement parks, and suburban backyards. (p. 270)

Further, by insisting on its own obsolescence, technology disguises its origin. By constantly ignoring its own past, it threatens the individual's (user's) stock of knowledge. It creates a cyborglike dependency based on brittle circuitry which constantly reminds us that a total collapse of the present moment awaits . . . leaving the self existentially alone but scarcely equipped to take advantage of existentialism's promise (Stretch, 1967).

Hypertechnology Scene #4

Due to the number of times your mouse has fallen off its pad and onto the floor, your double click button needs a veritable four, eight, or ten count series of extra hard knocks to be properly recognized by the software running on your machine.

Power Issues

Hypertechnology subtly fronts for power and control issues among administration, staff, faculty, students, and clients. Technology by itself, Heidegger asserted, is rarely the issue. Technology can be trivially seen to include both end-seeking human activity and the use of equipment, tools, and machines to achieve those ends to control nature (Ferre, 1995, p. 65).

Hypertechnology Scene #5

Someone in administration decided you can't use your word processor graphics package, database, stat package, or spreadsheet anymore. . .

The problem of technology, according to Heidegger, is that before one can attempt to control nature, there must first be an inclination to improve efficiency, the technological a priori, which is not in itself a machine or anything overtly technological, but rather a pragmatic motive. But this is only part of the problem, according to Ferre (1995):

> When we start to wonder whether modern technology is out of our control, we exhort ourselves to "master" it. But if the technological a priori is the will to mastery itself, then our firmest determinations will merely pour fuel on the allconsuming flames of the modern technological phenomenon. The more we will to master it, the more it masters us through the technological quality of our act of willing. (pp. 66-67)

Ontologically, Heidegger claims that regardless of the type of object (technology) under discussion, the very status of object itself—something standing firmly over and against us—just being what it is—is lost by the technological reduction of existence to those things waiting to be used (Ferre, 1995, p. 67). This sort of instrumentality in social work drives out every other possibility of being and revealing, undercutting the very foundation of social work as a profession.

The Creation of Complexity

Hypertechnology in social work creates pseudocomplexity out of what was once simplicity. Studies have shown that three-dimensional graphics packages can lead individuals (users) to generate totally incorrect conclusions out of material which experts agree had barely enough value to merit a single dimension to begin with (Tufte, 1983).

Hypertechnology Scene #6

> By the way, all of your overhead transparencies and handouts will need to be reconfigured to the landscape (sideways) mode as telecommunications people tell you that television is oriented sideways. When you work online you'll need to reorient all this material.

Research on social work journals (Orme and Combs-Orme, 1986) finds that increasing statistical power via hypertechnology does not produce better social work knowledge. In fact, it heightens the probability of trivial, pop-sociologistic projects that contribute nothing to our knowledge base (Kreuger, 1993). The editorial boards of major social work journals are not protecting us from these suspect studies. According to Pardeck (1992):

> Again, if the scholarship attainments of editorial board members are questionable and if many have never contributed to the social work or social science literatures, how can the articles published in social work journals reviewed and approved by such board members have credibility? (p. 531)

WHAT SHOULD WE DO
AS EDUCATORS/PRACTITIONERS?

We agree with Agger (1991) that practice, whether as education or clinical/field, should not be seen so much as transmission of information as construction and conversation. To be effective it must be thoroughly textual and dialogical. Thus, it follows that for us to understand and responsibly incorporate hypertechnology we must first develop a narrative that demystifies those precious objects which too often are held up in sacred and privileged ways by those who worship at the altar of efficiency only. We propose that a set of narrative standards offered by Hauerwas and Jones (1989) be at the heart of our model of technofreedom. Any narrative that we adopt, or allow to adopt us, will have to display:

1. the power to release us from destructive alternatives;
2. ways of seeing through current distortions;
3. room to keep us from having to resort to violence; and
4. a sense for the tragic: how meaning transcends power. (p. 185)

Just as Agger (1991) recognizes that every reading changes a text, so too must every technoencounter (usage) be seen to change hypertechnology. Technology cannot be fully understood as a narrative apart from the interpretive practices of those who engage it. Technology can only have meaning in specific places; it is given its sense only when individuals (users) participate in it as fully privileged narrative partners. We agree with Fisher (1992) that we must create new narratives that free us from technobondage:

> The narrative paradigm presupposes a world constituted by stories and the view that no form of discourse is to be privileged over others because its form is predominantly argumentative. No matter how strictly a case is argued, theologically, scientifically, philosophically, or legally, it will always be a story. (p. 209)

A genuine technofreedom from the all-encompassing power of hypertechnology requires that people know how to access and freely use it in nondominating ways. They must understand technology poststructurally, by recognizing that every use strongly contributes to a technology's meaning, just as every narrative is an argument for one or another state of affairs. Using technology is not a neutral reliance upon this or that piece of office equipment. Technology is not part of nature in the sense that it has meaning apart from the sweat expended to formulate and interpret it. Dialogue and discourse and eventually technofreedom depend on this understanding of technology's contingent, sometimes capricious character (Agger, 1991).

Our preferred technofreedom depends on a critical awareness of how to engage technology posttechnically and deconstructively, understanding its potential for being reformulated and hence ultimately liberating for the individual. Technology is not just units of equipment; it is also the lives it scripts for individuals—the lives they live by their own example. Without this sort of understanding, social workers will remain in the thrall of technologies that appear to have arrived as if by epiphany, having neither history nor social or cultural significance. This is the most dangerous situation of all—the ignorant capitulation to scientism, technicism, and busy consumerism of the marketplace.

With Derrida (1976), we insist that technology is undecidable in the sense that it conceals conflicts within it between different authorial voices. Technology must be seen as a contested terrain in the sense that what it appears to "say" on the surface cannot be understood without reference to the concealments and contextualizations of meaning going on simultaneously to mark its significance (e.g., use of specialized jargon). These concealments and contextualizations might be viewed as the assumptions that every technology makes in presuming that it will be understood.

IS COMMUNITY POSSIBLE?

Given these conditions, how are we to respond? How do we conceptualize and then respond to hypertechnological domination?

Following a model of postmodernism developed by Hassan (1982, p. 250), the authors have conceptualized a technology continuum that ranges from the current situation of hypertechnological bondage to a condition of hypertechnological freedom.

HYPERTECHNOLOGICAL BONDAGE	HYPERTECHNOLOGICAL FREEDOM
Form (conjunctive, closed)	Antiform (disjunctive, open)
Purpose	Play
Design	Chance
Hierarchy	Anarchy
Mastery/Logos	Exhaustion/Silence
Finished work	Process/Happening
Distance	Proximity
Creation/Totalization	Decreation/Deconstruction
Synthesis	Antithesis
Presence	Absence
Centering	Dispersal
Master Code	Idiolect
Origin/Cause	Difference/Trace
Determinacy	Indeterminacy

The following recommendations maintain the social work perspective that practice and education for practice take place within the sustaining tradition of the person-in-situation configuration. If technology best serves those ends, then we encourage its use. But the basic social work helping paradigm of enhancing social functioning by emphasizing change opportunities in a unique person-in-situation configuration should serve as the criterion against which to judge the value of our tools. Effective practice, in our view, demands that change and cure be sustained through interpersonal relationships. Here we present our recommendations for policy and practice:

1. We need to develop and legitimize informal *"Gemeinschaft-like"* groups that are relatively free from bureaucratic, technological intervention—during coffee breaks, at lunch, in the rest room, and during lulls in routine office work *(play, anarchy, and chance)*.

2. Erving Goffman (1959) suggested that individuals function within a framework of "fronts," or interactive spaces we may choose to hide within where a protective front operates within the parameters of an "official self," while keeping intact that which is really felt or believed *(silence, deconstruction, and idiolect)*. This needs to be encouraged.

3. Likewise, individuals possess an *Umwelt*, a psychological space where personal security and feelings of well-being can flourish (Goffman, 1959). An individual defines his or her territory, which then functions as a moving bubble of security (desk space, bathroom stall, "safe distance") and becomes a sacred domain *(antithesis, dispersal)*.

4. Technical jargon should be kept to a minimum and where possible translated into ordinary language. We need to prevent technological "subuniverses of meaning" from dominating the rest of our experience *(absence)*. We need to limit technospeak (Karger and Kreuger, 1988) or at least develop a set of enabling translation rules from the nonordinary language of technology into ordinary everyday vernacular *(idiolect)*.

5. No policy, program, or office activity should be undertaken unless it can be demonstrated to advance the interests of at least one social worker or client while harming no one *(indeterminacy)*.

6. All those affected by policies regarding technology should be encouraged to participate in the decision-making process so that monolithic office structures do not concentrate power in the hands of a few technical specialists *(open, disjunctive)*.

7. Those who possess insufficient technical skills should be given the choice to receive fully compensated technical training during working hours, or the opportunity to migrate to a nonautomated position with equality of remuneration *(process, happening)*.

8. Social work educators should demand free public access to the entire assemblage of hypermodern technology and free public terminals available and accessible to all without regard to their posi-

tion in various national and international marketplaces *(dispersal, difference)*.

9. Continued dialogue, discourse, and debate through traditional or specialized national forums in social work on the consequences of technology for the natural environment *(overcomes silence)*.

10. Issues of civil liberties, rights to privacy, and rights to intellectual property (Agre and Rotenberg, 1998), all need to be revisited and opened for debate *(difference, trace)*.

11. Professional boards and oversight committees associated with standards, licensing, and codes of ethics should demand a focus on achieving more humane outcomes, not just more equipment *(deconstruction)*.

12. Caution is urged in social work education against using faculty to broadcast outward from central studios. Our laboratory is in the community, not in our offices. We recommend more faculty outreach for on-site instruction in live practice settings such as hospices, hospitals, and neighborhood locales, jails, or homeless shelters to illustrate real-time, real-situation intervention *(proximity)*.

Chapter 5

Social Work Education: From Metanarrative to Curricular Variety

Within the context of college and university settings, social work education degree programs span the past century. As they continue to develop in the midst of the present postmodern era, ongoing opportunities and challenges must be faced. It remains to be seen whether the opportunities outweigh the challenges but, given the history of social work education, there may be more of the latter than the former. In this chapter several of the educational issues of a curricular and contextual nature are identified and discussed. As a segue to examining these issues, however, it is helpful to briefly review several of the defining events that have shaped the state of social work education as it now exists.

HISTORICAL BACKGROUND

The first training programs in social work at the university level were established around the beginning of the twentieth century at universities in major urban areas such as New York, Chicago, Boston, and St. Louis. To assess the level of professionalism of both practice and education by the second decade of the new century, a distinguished medical educator was invited to a major conference to speak about the question of whether social work met the criteria of being a legitimate profession. The answer provided by Abraham Flexner (1915) was that it did not. This led to an energetic but frantic effort on the part of practitioners and educators to rethink the nature of the profession and the state of education for practice. By 1919 it was clear that social work education was beginning to achieve a higher level of organizational sophistication when the Association of Training Schools for Professional Social Work (ATSPSW) was created with seventeen charter members (Austin, 1997). The new association represented both undergraduate and graduate programs but took the strong position that only two-year graduate programs provided professional training. Undergraduate programs were seen as providing an education at the preprofessional level. Thus appeared the first strain between the two levels, which persists to this day.

Also during the early decades of the century there arose two competing curricular models, particularly at the graduate level. One would emphasize a social reform mission based on the conviction that it was necessary to improve society in order to benefit individuals and families who were outside the mainstream. The other model centered on direct service and treatment to individuals and families on a case-by-case basis. In the main the latter model prevailed, since most students drawn to the new training programs were women who were either volunteers or employees of agencies providing services of this type. This model ushered in the practice methods of casework, group work, and community organization. In 1929 a meeting took place attended by social agency administrators, practitioners, and educators, called the Milford Conference (NASW, 1974). At this meeting it was affirmed that even though there were methods, all three types of practice possessed an underlying common and generic foundation of knowledge, values, and skills.

By 1942 the strain between undergraduate and graduate education was so pronounced that undergraduate programs formed their own organization, the National Association of Schools of Social Administration (NASSA). Its purpose was to improve the quality and enhance the status of undergraduate education. By that time education at this level was seen mainly as preparing students to work in the public sector. It was not until 1952, with the formation of the Council on Social Work Education (CSWE), that the two associations disbanded and all of social work education came under the purview of a single body. However, the tension between the two levels remained pronounced throughout the first half of the century and became more distinct with the Hollis-Taylor report in 1951 (Hollis and Taylor, 1951). In unambiguous language this report stated that two-year graduate programs provided the only professional training for social workers and it reaffirmed the multiple methods of casework, group work, and community organization. It was not until 1974 that the CSWE began to accredit undergraduate programs and legitimated their efforts for training at the beginning professional level.

A certain comfort level remained among graduate social work educators up through the decades of the 1940s and 1950s with the casework, group work, and community approaches. Threading throughout the curricula of all social work education programs of those times was an organizing paradigm, or what postmodernists now call a metanarrative. The metanarrative during this time was the Freudian psychoanalytic one, which provided a set of concepts and a theoretical foundation for understanding the human psyche and resultant behavior and the social interactions induced by it.

Both the social work education and practice communities became theoretical prisoners of the psychoanalytic model. However, during the mid- and late 1960s and early 1970s there appeared some cracks in the pedagogical and practical utility of the model. The War on Poverty called to the attention of the entire country as well as to that of professional practitioners and educators the necessity to move beyond a theoretical foundation that was basically intra-psychic and at times interpersonal in nature. It became evident that larger social structural conditions and inequalities might need to be remedied in order to provide the context for the improved functioning of individuals and families. The central insight of the emerging approach, or metanarrative, was that large numbers of persons were being denied access to the opportunity structures in employment, education, and economic assets. If this were true, then the psychoanalytic paradigm was irrelevant as an underpinning to professional social work education. The final nail in the coffin of the psychoanalytic model was driven with the advent of the community mental health movement in the early 1970s. The notion of community-centered and community-based treatment for mental illness required new conceptualizations that ranged far beyond the changing of intrapsychic dynamics. For practitioners within these new approaches it became necessary to learn more about the dynamics of individuals, families, and groups as well as organizations and communities. The target of intervention, or client, was not always the person but larger social arrangements.

Thus the comfort of the psychoanalytic metanarrative was abandoned in favor of a variety of behavioral and social science ones. The new metanarrative had a variety of names, but the two appearing most frequently in the social work literature were social systems theory and ecological theory.

It is difficult to determine when a profession is shedding one metanarrative or foundation theory for a replacement one as a basis for organizing practitioner behavior. Both psychoanalytic theory and systems/ecological theory did serve to provide a conceptual lens to understand the human and social realities under consideration. Both were also very influential as frameworks in developing curricula at the BSW and MSW program levels. These metanarratives enabled students and practitioners to assess, plan strategies for change, carry them out, and then evaluate how successful they were. These are now being abandoned, and the new era in which social work education and practice finds itself is flirting with a number of replacement perspectives. The most frequently cited ones are postmodernism, social constructionism, feminist theory, existentialism, critical theory, and hermeneutics. These all differ from both psychoanalysis and systems/ecological theory in one main respect.

The older theories were used in a top-down fashion in that they were overlaid as a conceptual lens and applied to the reality being studied. Postmodernism, social constructionism, and the others are bottom-up in that the perspective used to understand a reality is created, arises, and is fashioned by the reality itself. Each of the new perspectives begins with a belief that objective reality does not exist which precludes belief in a metanarrative or theory.

Within this chapter there will be an examination of several issues within social work education centering on curriculum, faculty, students, and program context. These issues can best be understood by remembering that social work education is now rudderless and without a metanarrative to guide it. The absence of such a paradigmatic foundation goes a long way in explaining the wide variation in curricular patterns within the rapidly expanding social work education community. However, before examining areas of concern it should be noted that the social work education establishment has made great strides.

A SUCCESS STORY

To the uninformed and casual observer of developments and trends in higher education in the United States, it would appear that social work education is one of the major success stories. This is particularly evident when quantitative data are considered, but less so from a qualitative perspective. From the quantitative point of view it is striking that over the past few decades the number of social work programs on college and university campuses has more than doubled. In addition, each year approximately ten or more programs at both the BSW and MSW levels achieve candidacy status, which is the category that immediately precedes full accreditation. All social work education programs are under the auspices of the CSWE, which is legally sanctioned to conduct reviews and render accreditation decisions. In October 1998, as shown in Table 5.1, 593 programs at both levels had achieved full accreditation from the CSWE or were in the candidacy stage of the accreditation process, which precedes initial accreditation (source: personal communication from CSWE, October 1998). Based on the number of social work education programs at that time, it is likely that within the first years of the twenty-first century that the number of accredited social work education programs will be in the range of 625 to 650. This phenomenal growth was accompanied by programs achieving

TABLE 5.1. Social Work Education Programs in the United States (October, 1998)

	Baccalaureate Level	Master's Level	All Programs
Full Accreditation	412	128	540
Candidacy Status	33	20	53
Total Programs	445	148	593

independent or autonomous organizational status within their respective institutions, particularly graduate ones. There are indications, however, that as institutions strive to cut administrative costs many social work programs will be absorbed into larger academic units. This has already happened to several schools of social work in prestigious universities and it is likely to continue with others. Interestingly, the same pattern has not appeared with undergraduate programs. In many instances when an undergraduate program located in another unit achieves full accreditation, it shortly is able to acquire university support for a separate social work department. As a general rule undergraduate social work education programs in smaller colleges appear to have more stature than do graduate programs in larger universities.

As programs have proliferated, a concomitant increase has occurred in the number of social work students enrolled and seeking degrees. In November 1997 the CSWE, which annually gathers statistics from all programs, reported 83,615 full- and part-time undergraduate and master's students enrolled in the programs that submitted data (CSWE, 1997). During that year these students were taught by 6,469 faculty. In the early years of the next century it is likely that social work students will number in excess of 100,000 and faculty over 7,000, given the rate at which new programs are accredited. A reasonable prediction is that by then social work education programs, students, and faculty might make up about 2 percent of the entire higher education enterprise.

Consistent with the growth of social work education programs, the employment demand for professionally trained social work practitioners has remained strong. The fields of practice that have traditionally employed large numbers of social workers, such as family service, health, mental health, and child welfare, continue to do so. With the introduction of the managed care movement in the health field and the opening up of new employment opportunities such as in occupational social work, the job market for social workers will remain healthy.

No definitive data exists on the actual number of professionally trained social workers in the United States. The major professional association for social workers, the National Association of Social Workers (NASW), in 1998 reported 152,425 active paid-up members (source: personal communication from NASW, November 1998). This is not an accurate measurement of the number of professionally trained and actively employed social workers, since it is well known and commonly accepted that the majority of those with professional degrees do not become members of NASW. Over the past decade both baccalaureate and master's social work education programs have annually awarded an average of 10,000 degrees. It is reasonable to assume, therefore, that there are at least 250,000 to 300,000 professionally trained social workers in the United States.

After casual review it appears, therefore, that given the apparent success of social work in the higher education community, along with the large number of social work practitioners who find gainful employment, social work education is the picture of health. And by these measures it can rightfully take credit for progress in those areas. However, long-standing conditions and issues urge some caution before declaring it an unqualified success. Some of these issues have persisted for decades and exist below the current collective consciousness of the educational community. They are present but are glossed over. Nevertheless, they have an impact on both the structure and curricular patterns of social work education. Along with long-standing subsurface issues contemporary conditions exist that are cause for some concern. The concerns are serious ones, dealing with issues such as whether the social work curriculum possesses conceptual "clarity and coherence" and whether it is indeed a program of professional preparation that is inchoate in nature and unable to prepare practitioners for the future trends facing society (Bisno and Cox, 1997). In this chapter both long-standing and current conditions within social work education are examined and the implications are discussed.

BSW AND MSW CURRICULAR TENSION

When social work education is subjected to an examination that delves below its documented numerical successes in establishing programs and attracting students, and begins to study long-standing conditions and issues, there appear to be areas of concern. These conditions are now part of the educational infrastructure and in daily pedagogical efforts and activities tend to fall below the level of awareness of administrators, faculty, and students. For at least half a century, as pointed out by Dinerman (1994), there has been tension and disagreement about whether there should be two social work degrees or one. She points out that prior to 1950, undergraduate and graduate programs existed in a state of reciprocal uneasiness. Then, in 1951, a report by a group of distinguished social work educators unambiguously declared that the only legitimate preparation for professional social workers should consist of two years of graduate study (Hollis and Taylor, 1951). Twenty years would pass before the CSWE began to officially accredit undergraduate programs in 1971, which launched the phenomenal growth in BSW programs over the following twenty-five years.

The uneasiness identified half a century ago between BSW and MSW programs has persisted to the present time, although it tends to remain in the background and is rarely discussed openly. It is not an insignificant issue and resembles a century-long conceptual rollercoaster. For the first half of the century both degree levels existed without demonstrable tension, with the graduate-level occupying the bellwether role. Following the advent of the Hollis-Taylor report, official policy declared graduate level education as the only legitimate preparation of professional social workers. For the next quarter century tension ran high between advocates of the two levels until CSWE officially began to accredit BSW programs in the 1970s. From that date on the balance of power in the social work education community swung away from the graduate level toward one of dynamic tension. Open conflict as well subsurface tension appeared throughout social work education. Frequently, divisions appeared between faculty in programs offering both levels of degrees. Faculty in graduate programs seemed to hold more stature than their undergraduate colleagues. It was not uncommon for graduate programs to receive higher personnel and budgetary resources. As an example of interprogram disparity, the official CSWE accreditation standard for faculty size recommends one faculty person for every twelve students in graduate programs. It recommends one faculty member for every twenty-five students at the undergraduate level. As far as can be determined, no body of research findings or compelling conceptual formulations supports this policy. It is an artifact of a policy enacted during the period when graduate faculty held more power in the CSWE than those at the undergraduate level. This era witnessed the appearance and influence of special interest groups in social work education and the beginning of a decision-making pattern in which political considerations played a major role.

Clear consensus and agreement has never been reached about the need, the logical connectiveness, and what the essential focus should be at the two levels of social work education. In terms of need, the Great Society era of the early 1960s opened up a vast array of social service positions, most of which were filled by untrained personnel. The social work community, particularly the NASW, advocated vigorously in the late 1960s and early 1970s to increase baccalaureate-educated social work practitioners to fill positions that were being occupied by nontrained persons. This was a critical juncture in the historical development of social work practice and education. The choice was whether to create an undergraduate professional degree to meet the critical employment need or to launch a massive increase of the number of graduate programs. The choice to support an increase in undergraduate over graduate education was not made dispassionately and in a climate of reasoned debate. Rather, the proponents in the BSW camp advocated strongly on their own behalf and, with the support of the NASW, were able to carry the day. CSWE quickly came on board and began accrediting BSW programs in 1971. Over the next twenty-five years an average of sixteen new BSW programs has been accredited every year, to the present level of 412 programs (see Table 5.1). The faculty and leadership within the graduate ranks were not happy with the speed at which undergraduate programs proliferated, which created a tension between the two levels that still exists. The deans/directors of MSW programs have their own professional association that is not affiliated with the BSW administrator's group. Both groups meet separately at different sites and have no official organizational mechanism to engage in sustained collaborative efforts.

THE BSW CURRICULAR CONUNDRUM

With the reality of two officially sanctioned levels of social work education facing faculty, there was a distinct climate of ambivalence and indecisiveness about the nature of the curriculum to be offered at both. It seemed clear that two curricular development options could be pursued. The first was the establishment of a continuum of social work education beginning with the associate degree level, moving up through the baccalaureate and master's levels, and ending with the doctorate. The education continuum spanning the BSW and MSW levels was widely discussed at professional meetings, but the idea always seemed to fall short of meeting acceptable pedagogical attributes. Some of the characteristics of a continuum were articulated by Gross (1992) and included, among others, separate content foci at both levels and nonrepetitive content at the higher one. The graduate level should contain more complex content and both levels were to be compatible with distinct employment opportunities in the world of practice. It has never been possible to clearly document that the four characteristics were met in the BSW-MSW continuum.

As thinking about the two levels of social work education evolved, it eventuated in an official enunciation of distinctive BSW and MSW curricular foci. These are articulated in the most recent accreditation standards (CSWE, 1994a, b) and curriculum policy statements (CSWE, 1992a, b). After months of deliberation it was declared and officially sanctioned by the CSWE that BSW-level social work education would have as its central mission the preparation of students for general social work practice. This meant that they would be provided with educational preparation to enable them to practice with individuals, families, groups, organizations, and communities. The mission of MSW graduate programs was to focus on educational preparation for an advanced level of social work practice in an area of concentration.

Based on the different purpose and objectives of BSW and MSW programs, there is a serious question about the decision to focus at the first level on the broadest and most generalized scope of human reality and at the second on the most specific and concentrated. The first two years in BSW programs are organized around the acquisition of a liberal arts education, which is considered essential to and supportive of the professional social work courses offered in the junior and senior years. In the last two years of the professional program the content areas that BSW-level students are expected to master is extremely broad in scope. It is questionable whether a sound mastery of all the content areas can be obtained in this relatively short period of time. Table 5.2 describes seven categories of educational content to be presented including the enormous scope of information to be covered within each category.

Each of the seven categories in Table 5.2 for which BSW students are expected not only to develop intellectual mastery but practice skills as well includes a large number of content areas. In this regard it is illustrative to examine the levels of human systems for which students are officially expected to develop practice competencies. Students must acquire knowledge about normal functioning, knowledge about abnormal functioning, and skills to bring about change in each level. It can easily be seen that functioning within each level can only be understood as interactive with levels below and above it.

Thus, to understand organizational functioning it is necessary to examine how the groups within it influence internal dynamics, and how the community environment impacts on organizational functioning. Also, each level has a body of research findings that is important to master. There is an equal degree of informational scope within the other categories of social problems, diverse populations, practice roles, change technologies, practice settings, and body of theories. It is unreasonable to expect that BSW students with two years of social work courses will acquire the proficiency to engage in professional practice of such complexity. In fact, given this scope and complexity, it is more reasonable to offer this content at the graduate MSW level and adopt a more focused mission at the undergraduate BSW level. In the judgment of many it is not a feasible educational objective to expect students in a BSW program covering two years of social work course work to master the scope of content described above and acquire professional practice competency.

The counterargument to the assertion just presented is that BSW-level students are taught a generalist approach to practice that is applicable to all situations. This approach involves skills of observation and data gathering, problem assessment, planning, change intervention activities, and evaluation of efforts. It is also

TABLE 5.2. The Scope of Content in BSW Social Work Programs

Content Categories	Scope of Content
Levels of Systems	Includes information about persons, groups, families, organizations, and communities. Each level of systems must include research findings and theories about normal and abnormal functioning and the functional interdependency between the levels.
Human and Social Problems and Needs	Each level of systems is characterized by unique forms of functioning and possesses idiosyncratic problem configurations. In addition, economic, social, and cultural problems that impact each of the levels must be understood.
Vulnerable and Diverse Populations	At each system level there are variable societal groups for which social work has special responsibility. These include the poor, elderly, children, mentally ill, abused, and incarcerated, among others.
Change Methods, Strategies, and Technologies	There is a vast body of research about the variable modes of change efforts to be differentially applied to the system levels, diverse populations, and problem configurations.
Eclectic Range of Theory	To practice effectively with a range of systems; with variable complex social problems, with diverse populations, and applying multiple methods requires acquaintance with and ability to select from a large body of relevant theories.
Practice Roles	The generalist perspective requires the application of multiple practice roles and behaviors including case manager, broker, advocate, teacher, evaluator, enabler, mediator, consultant, administrator, community organizer, counselor, and caregiver, among others.
Practice Settings	It is expected that BSW education prepares students for beginning professional practice across the entire panoply of human service organizations. Major ones include family services, child welfare, health, mental health, aging, corrections, and occupational social work.

obvious that this approach has such a high level of abstraction that it could apply to all problem-solving activities across all professions and is not unique to social work. Those who have studied the generalist approach have concluded that confusion occurs about what it means (Landon, 1995) and that it implies "superman" competencies whereby the social worker does "anything for anyone" (Pardeck et al., 1998). There are no definitional and conceptual boundaries for the generalist curricular model, and it clearly is difficult to logically defend it as appropriate and relevant as the central focus of baccalaureate social work education. A very distinguished social work educator (Hartman, 1983) has pointed out that it is reasonable to reverse the generalist-specialist curricular arrangement. According to her, BSW programs could provide concrete knowledge and skills to be applied in specific situations. MSW programs would then offer a wider and more varied range of knowledge and skills at a higher level of abstraction and applicable to a broader and more complex range of situations.

CONCENTRATIONS WITHOUT BOUNDARIES

Originating with an official curriculum policy authorized by the CSWE in 1969, all graduate social work education programs were expected to offer a concentration. As specified at the time, the most notable characteristic of a concentration was to be a distinctive pattern of instruction organized around a specific range of professional practice roles and functions. Each program was given complete responsibility and freedom to design concentrations and their constituent courses. The only requirements specified by the CSWE were that concentrations be relevant to the mission of social work, and that suitable roles and functions be available for those who complete them. In the ensuing years the fundamental policy about concentrations has not changed in that programs continue to have complete freedom to select whatever concentrations they wish. Thus they remain without conceptual boundaries and in this regard are similar to the generalist focus at the undergraduate level. This apparently limitless and expansive curricular scope is characteristic of the entire profession of social work, which has never established a definitive conceptual and practice niche within the field of the social and helping professions.

Shortly after the establishment of concentrations it was possible to discern overall models among the array that had been created by various programs. Meinert's (1979) study, which was subsequently replicated by Brooks (1982), identified five patterns of concentrations. These were: (1) "traditional," consisting of casework, group work, or community organization methods; (2) "individualized," consisting of a set of individually selected courses; (3) "dual track," which focused on either direct (micro) or indirect (macro) intervention skills; (4) "specific," which centered on a unique and identifiable field of practice, population group, or problem area; and (5) "matrix," which combined two or more variables such as field of practice and level of intervention. In reviewing all the concentrations from graduate programs in 1998 using this five-feature model, it became evident that it was not currently valid and that it could no longer be reliably applied. A major reason for this was that many programs have included additional dimensions in their concentrations. Several programs had a matrix model involving two levels of intervention (micro and macro) in several fields of practice. However, then they would add what were variously referred to as a focus, an emphasis, a dimension, an incorporation, an area, or a theme, among others. Thus, for example, a student might learn direct service intervention skills in the field of mental health with an emphasis on ethnic minority populations. This is indeed a logical combination, but is unlikely that the concentration design would be able to adhere to the required accreditation standards. These require that the concentration (1) be anchored in a liberal arts perspective and the professional foundation (generalist approach); (2) be built on relevant theories; (3) contain educational content specific to the concentration; and (4) provide practicum opportunities that logically match the several dimensions of the concentration. It is not likely that complex multidimensional concentrations can possess a high degree of fidelity to all four requirements.

Perhaps the major area of concern about concentrations is their embeddedness in information about fields of practice and the placement of students in practica organized by fields of practice. Social work education statistics (CSWE, 1997) document that students are assigned practicum settings in fourteen major fields of practice. It is reasonable to expect that students in a specific concentration in a specific field of practice would engage in practice skills and behaviors that are unique to it. As convincingly shown by Raymond, Teare, and Atherton (1996) in a large study of professional social workers, there are no meaningful differences in tasks performed across fields of practice. It would be more reasonable to have MSW students learn advanced skills and techniques that are applicable in a variety of fields. Those who hold this view advocate the advanced generalist as the focus for MSW-level education.

CONTEXTUAL ISSUES

Educators and administrators should be concerned about certain conditions in spite of the numerical success of social work education at both levels as evidenced by the dramatic increase in the number of programs, students, and faculty. Many of these conditions are not included by the CSWE as part of the accreditation review process. For example, before advancing to the status of candidate for accreditation a petitioning program must document that a need exists for its graduates. If it is unable to do so to the satisfaction of the CSWE, it is not granted candidacy status. However, once candidacy status is achieved and following initial accreditation this question is never again raised. After examining the low number of students and small number of degrees awarded by many programs, it is reasonable to conclude that many currently accredited programs are not meeting a documented need. CSWE data for 1997 reveals that fifty BSW programs awarded ten or fewer degrees and several awarded only one, two, or three. It would be difficult to argue that these programs are meeting community needs. If indeed a community need is great, then these programs are underproducing graduates to fill it. The other side of the coin is that they may be awarding only a small number of BSW degrees because there is no community need for them. The CSWE takes no deaccreditation action against these low-producing BSW programs. Thus there currently exist many accredited BSW programs for which there is no documented need. A similar disparity exists between high- and low-degree-producing graduate programs. In 1997 the average number of MSW degrees awarded by all programs reporting to the CSWE (N = 115) was 130. Table 5.3 exhibits the top five and low five MSW degree-producing programs (CSWE, 1997). Again, the question must be raised as to whether a need actually exists in those communities where MSW programs award so few degrees.

This situation demonstrates a characteristic of the CSWE that can be viewed either as positive or negative according to which perspective is adopted. It has absolutely no control over broad directions, conditions, and developments beyond the level of features intrinsic to individual programs. It limits itself to the accreditation process program by program, and does not purport to examine and have an impact on social work education issues on a national level. An organizational void exists in this area and issues of national import are ignored. In the sections that follow, several noncurricular issues of a contextual nature are examined. Those responsible for social work education programs should be concerned about all of these issues, since they have an effect on quality in the educational process.

TABLE 5.3. Programs Awarding Highest and Lowest Numbers of MSW Degrees (1997)

Most Awarded	Fewest Awarded
626—Fordham	12—North Dakota
459—New York University	12—Gallaudet
386—Columbia	16—Portland State
367—Maryland	17—Boise State
347—Rutgers	21—Nevada/Reno

PROGRAM SELECTIVITY

One of the issues of concern is the results of the admissions process for social work education programs in terms of whether they admit students with the highest academic potential. The literature appears to lack discussion about the decision process by which graduate social work education programs select students for admission. Professional as well as conventional wisdom asserts that graduate programs desire to admit intelligent, motivated, and well-prepared students. All programs as a requirement for accreditation must have written admission policies and procedures to ensure that only the persons best qualified to become professional social workers are admitted. It is mandatory that programs select the persons who exhibit the most promise of successfully achieving the professional education goals that have been established. Therefore, the percentage of students accepted from the pool of those considered for admission is certainly one measure of a program's quality. In fall 1997, for the 111 MSW programs submitting data to the CSWE, the national average was 60.5 percent official admissions from the total pool of those who had applied for full-time enrollment and were considered (CSWE, 1997) This means that six out every ten persons who applied and were considered for admission and enrollment were accepted. The acceptance rates for those seeking part-time admission and for students applying for advanced standing was even higher than those for full-time programs. The acceptance rate for part-time students was 66.2 percent; for advanced standing students it was 67.7 percent (advanced standing students are ones with BSW degrees who complete the requirements for the MSW degree in approximately one calendar year). Whether this is high or low is a subjective judgment. However, within the 111 programs the pattern of acceptance variation was extreme, ranging from five programs that admitted under 25 percent of those who were considered and eight that admitted over 90 percent of those considered. Two programs admitted 100 percent of those considered for admission.

There is no official method for ranking MSW programs (Meinert, 1993; Kreuger, 1993). The CSWE has a curriculum policy statement and a manual of accreditation standards, both containing requirements to be met if programs are to achieve and maintain accredited status. Programs meeting the requirements in these materials have met specified minimal standards, but it is made clear that qualitative differences are not to be made or inferred by virtue of achieving accredited status. There have been numerous attempts to rank MSW programs, most often on the basis of subjective reputations, counting faculty publications and citations, library holdings, and funding patterns. None of these attempts have examined the variation in admissions or the extent to which applicants to programs actually register and enroll in programs following official acceptance.

A list was prepared of the top-ranked MSW programs by including those appearing most often in ten separate ranking studies. Nine of these made a composite ranking based on previously published reports that ranked schools of social work (Kirk and Corcoran, 1995). The tenth appeared in a recent ranking of professional schools by *U.S. News and World Report* (1998). From the ten separate rankings, thirty-five programs appeared most often and they arguably constitute the best of all the accredited MSW programs. Several variables were used among the ten rankings including reputational opinions, faculty publication counts, faculty citation counts, library resources, and funding patterns.

Within the thirty-five MSW programs an analysis of the rate at which applicants are accepted for admission reveals a wide pattern. Three of the programs accepted under 25 percent of those who were considered, while two programs had an acceptance rate of over 90 percent. For purposes of analysis, programs with acceptance rates of under 40 percent are categorized as very selective; 40.1 to 60 percent as selective; 60.1 to 75 percent as unselective; and 75.1 to 100 percent as very unselective. It is asserted that the rate at which programs accept students from the total who were considered for admission is a strong measure of the quality of the program. Low admission rates indicate a high level of quality and high admission rates a low level of quality. Why the admission rates among schools exhibit such wide variation can only be speculated about. One explanation could be that some programs set admission goals and admit students until the goal is achieved and thus become unselective and casual in decisions about applicants. A second reason might be that in some programs the acquisition of university budgetary resources is linked to enrollment and admissions standards are loose to ensure high enrollments. Third, some might be admitting a large number of students who have marginal academic performance in order to enroll persons with characteristics the program has deemed desirable. The percentages in Table 5.4 were derived from self-reported data submitted to the CSWE (CSWE, 1997).

TABLE 5.4. Acceptance Rates Among Thirty-Four Previously Top-Ranked MSW Programs

Very Selective	Selective
22.5%—North Carolina	42.3%—Hunter
23.3%—California/Berkeley	42.9%—Ohio State
24.3%—Illinois/Chicago	45.7%—University of Washington
30.7%—UCLA	47.6%—Wisconsin/Madison
36.3%—Chicago	54.8%—Boston College
40.0%—Minnesota/Minneapolis	56.1%—Wisconsin/Milwaukee
	58.3%—SUNY Albany
	59.6% Houston

Unselective	Very Unselective
60.3%—Pittsburgh	75.1%—Columbia
60.7%—Maryland	77.3%—Florida State
60.9%—Texas/Arlington	81.3%—Fordham
62.0%—Tennessee	81.4%—Texas/Austin
63.3%—Smith	81.5%—Denver
63.9%—Kansas	85.4%—Adelphi
66.5%—Boston University	87.2%—Washington U./St. Louis
67.2%—Illinois/Urbana	93.9%—Pennsylvania
69.4%—Southern California	96.0%—Case Western Reserve
69.9%—Bryn Mawr	
73.9%—Michigan	
74.1%—Virginia	

Note: One of the thirty-five top-ranked programs did not report data to CSWE.

TABLE 5.5. Most Selective and Least Selective MSW Programs by Percentage of Applicants Accepted from Those Considered for Admission

Most Selective Programs	Least Selective Programs
8.2%—San Francisco	85.4%—Adelphi
22.5%—North Carolina	87.2%—Washington/St. Louis
23.3%—California/Berkeley	90.1%—West Virginia
23.8%—Southern Connecticut	92.7%—Kentucky
24.3%—Illinois/Chicago	93.2%—Our Lady of the Lake
27.3%—Brigham Young	93.9%—Pennsylvania
28.0%—Widener	96.0%—Case Western Reserve
28.6%—East Carolina	97.3%—Howard
30.7%—UCLA	100.0%—Eastern Michigan
33.0%—New Mexico	100.0%—Walla Walla

The ten accredited MSW programs with the most professionally stringent record of acceptance decisions are listed in Table 5.5 paired with the ten having the least stringent record. The lowest rates of admissions are all 33 percent or less, and the highest rates are all 85 percent or more (CSWE, 1997). It should be of great concern to the CSWE that many programs have an inordinately high ratio of acceptances to applications from the perspective of student quality. Several programs on the list of least selective in student admissions regularly appear in the top ten of the highest-ranked schools of social work. Many of the schools that never garner high scores in social work education ranking studies appear to be more selective in admitting students than those who appear frequently among the top rankings. At least four of the schools with least selective admission acceptance records consistently appear in the top rankings as measured by faculty publications and reputational studies.

STUDENT PREFERENCE

The CSWE (1997) statistical data as reported by graduate programs reveals significant variation in the percentage of students who actually register and enroll from the pool of those who were granted admission. These data clearly demonstrate that in many programs students enroll at a much higher rate following acceptance than in others. For all 111 programs nationally in 1997 the average rate of enrollment to acceptance was 55.4 percent. In other words, a little over half of all students who are officially accepted by a program actually register and enroll in it. For students seeking enrollment on a part-time basis the rate was 77.1 percent and for advanced standing students it was 65.5 percent.

It is not clear why there is wide variation among programs in the full-time student category in terms of the number of those who actually register and enroll from the number who applied. It ranges from a high of 100 percent enrolled from those accepted to a low of 29.3 percent. For this analysis, programs that have an enrollment-to-acceptance rate of 80 percent or higher are considered as very preferred by applicants. Those with an enrollment-to-acceptance rate of 45 percent and under are considered of low preference by applicants. One of the reasons students enroll in a particular program is that it represents a highly valued career objective. Students may choose to enroll for other reasons including proximity to their community of residence, auspice of the institution such as religious/nonreligious or public/private, cost of tuition, perceived reputation of institution and faculty, educational focus, and availability of financial aid, among others. Using enrollment-to-acceptance rates as a measure of student preference, the programs that were most preferred and least preferred by students appear in Table 5.6. The assumption underlying the data is that comparisons can be made between most attractive and preferred and least attractive and preferred programs on the basis of the extent to which applicants actually enroll and register following their official acceptance. Note that over half of the programs in the least preferred category are from schools of social work which are typically ranked high and located in very prestigious universities.

FACULTY RESOURCE DISPARITY

In the two decades since 1975 when the CSWE began accrediting undergraduate social work education programs, they have become the

TABLE 5.6. Most Preferred and Least Preferred MSW Programs Based on Acceptance-to-Enrollment Rates

Most Preferred	Least Preferred
100.0%—Eastern Michigan	29.3%—Fordham
100.0%—South Florida	33.3%—Maine
100.0%—Nevada/Reno	33.6%—Wisconsin/Madison
97.2%—Chicago	33.6%—New York University
96.4%—Louisville	35.8%—Pennsylvania
94.3%—Loma Linda	38.5%—Simmons
92.0%—Southern University	38.5%—Loyola
89.8%—San Francisco	38.8%—West Virginia
87.2%—Nebraska	39.9%—Boston University
84.1%—Widener	40.0%—Augsburg
83.3%—Brigham Young	40.4%—Vermont
82.4%—Illinois/Chicago	40.5%—Salem College
81.8%—New Mexico	41.4%—Boston College
81.5%—Utah	42.2%—Denver
80.9%—Grand Valley	43.9%—Michigan State
80.0%—SUNY Buffalo	44.6%—Washington/St. Louis

largest component of the three levels of social work education (BSW, MSW, and PhD). In 1997 the CSWE reported there were 111 MSW and 400 BSW programs and 91 of these were in joint BSW/MSW organizational arrangements (the CSWE does not accredit programs at the doctoral level). It might be expected that the distribution of faculty resources between BSW and MSW programs would approach some level of proportionality. However, as shown in Table 5.7, faculty resources from programs submitting data to the CSWE in 1997 are skewed between the two. BSW programs constitute over 70 percent of the total number of programs at all levels yet only have 26.4 percent of the faculty.

TABLE 5.7. MSW and BSW Program Faculty Distribution (1997)

	Programs		Faculty	
Level	Number	Percentage	Number	Percentage
MSW Only	42	9.5	2079	30.6
MSW & BSW	90	20.4	2915	43.0
BSW Only	309	70.1	1788	26.4
	441	100.0	6782	100.0

The BSW programs submitting data for the CSWE 1997 statistical survey reported 26,145 students at the junior and senior levels. Students at these levels are considered to be in the professional component of their training and as having completed the major liberal arts require ments. In this same year MSW programs reported 23,247 full-time students. No ready explanation is evident for the disproportionality in the assignment of faculty resources between the two categories of students. Clearly there are more BSW programs and students, but they have significantly fewer faculty.

Official CSWE accreditation standards (CSWE, 1994a, 1994b) recommend a faculty-to-student ratio of 1.25 at the undergraduate level and 1:12 at the graduate level. Programs that exceed this standard would be viewed with concern by the accrediting organization and asked to undertake efforts to meet it as soon as practicable. The standards do not provide a rationale for why it is desirable to have these different faculty-to-student ratios at the two levels. A review of the social work literature did not locate studies about it or pedagogical discussions to support it. In the opinion of the authors it is a residual of the earlier conflict in social work education about whether undergraduate education possessed the same degree of legitimacy as graduate education. From earliest times the BSW degree was not accorded the same level of professional acceptability as the MSW. In the early and mid-1970s social service programs were proliferating at a rapid rate. As a result of the 1964 War on Poverty and the earlier launching by President Kennedy of the community mental health movement the infusion of resources from the federal government created many social service and mental health programs. Graduate-level social workers and professionally trained personnel in other human service areas were insufficient in number to staff the emergent programs. Undergraduate training programs in social work and human service generalists were seen as a solution to the rising need for "professional" personnel. However, within the graduate social work education establishment this development was not met with enthusiasm. The elevation of graduate education to a higher status than undergraduate education accounts for the continued disparity in many areas including the belief that MSW faculty-to-student ratios should be smaller than BSW ones.

Other disparities between BSW and MSW programs can be seen when the highest educational attainment of faculty and their salaries are examined (CSWE, 1997). The educational attainment of faculty in combined graduate/undergraduate programs is at a higher level than in undergraduate-only programs, as indicated in Table 5.8 (CSWE does not provide information about educational attainment for MSW-only programs).

There are more programs and students at the BSW level than at the MSW level, yet the BSW programs have the fewest faculty and their level of educational attainment is lower than that of their graduate colleagues. Since BSW faculty clearly have fewer doctorates it is reasonable to assume that graduate-only programs have a higher percentage of doctorates than MSW/joint programs. CSWE does not report educational attainment for graduate-only programs, only MSW/BSW joint ones. It is likely that the percentage of faculty with doctorates in graduate-only programs approaches 70 to 80 percent. There is also a wide salary differential for faculty and administrators within the two program levels. Classroom instructors in MSW/joint programs have an annual median salary of $46,734 per year while

TABLE 5.8. Highest Educational Attainment of BSW and MSW Program Faculty

	BSW		MSW	
Attainment	Number	Percentage	Number	Percentage
Master's (Social Work and Other)	1055	60.5	2185	46.6
Doctorate (Social Work and Other)	691	39.5	2507	53.4
Total	1746	100.0	4692	100.0

their colleagues in BSW programs earn a median salary of $37,000. The annual median salary for administrators in MSW/joint programs is $86,462 while for those in BSW programs it is $44,971. This is additional evidence that in social work education, graduate programs are valued much more highly than undergraduate ones.

GENDER AND DIVERSITY ISSUES

One of the most evident, but essentially unexamined, characteristics of social work education and practice is the numerical preponderance of women over men. Social work is among several occupations such as nurses, librarians, and elementary school teachers that have a majority of female members. Theorizing and systematic empirical research directed to explaining this situation or its impact on the profession is lacking. No accurate data exist about the number of professionally trained social work practitioners in the United States. The NASW is the organization representing the largest number of social workers in the country. The members of the association, limited to persons with either undergraduate or graduate degrees from accredited social work education programs, are women in overwhelming numbers. The most recent membership data report 119,990 dues-paying female members and 29,985 male members. This represents approximately an 8:2 ratio of women over men. In the future it is unquestionably true that women will continue to predominate numerically as evidenced by the number of men and women who are currently enrolled in social work education programs. The most recent enrollment data (CSWE, 1997) for men and women in BSW and MSW programs, as displayed in Table 5.9, suggests that in the coming years the percentage of women in the profession will increase beyond 80 percent given that female enrollment exceeds that level.

TABLE 5.9. Student Enrollment by Gender (1997)

Program Level	Male		Female	
	Number	Percentage	Number	Percentage
BSW	3,530	13.5	22,615	86.5
MSW	3,554	16.2	18,981	83.8
Both Levels	7,194	14.7	41,596	85.3

The current enrollment by gender in social work education programs is consistent with degrees awarded in 1996-1997. In that year 13.9 percent of BSW degrees were awarded to men and 86.1 percent to women. At the MSW level 16.2 percent of the degrees were awarded to men and 83.8 percent to women.

In recent years women have increasingly moved into major administrative positions in social work education programs and now constitute a clear majority of the occupants of those positions. This was established by having two persons with social work training independently review the names of all the deans, directors, and chairs that are listed in the 1998 CSWE directory of social work education programs in the United States (CSWE, 1998). This included programs already accredited as well as those in candidacy status at both BSW and MSW levels. Several names were eliminated from consideration since it was not possible to determine the gender. The two reviewers agreed on the gender of the remaining names in 99.5 percent of the judgments, which indicates a high degree of reliability. Table 5.10 presents social work education administrators by program level and gender. The number of women social work education administrators has increased over the past two decades and is expected to continue to climb at a steady pace.

The gender distribution of social work faculty follows the same pattern as with administrators in that the majority are women. This is true for both BSW and MSW levels. For programs at all levels, accredited and in candidacy, there are a total of 585 administrators of which 57.9 percent are women and 42.1 percent are men. In this regard women clearly outnumber men in positions where more

TABLE 5.10. Gender of Social Work Education Administrators

Program Level	Male		Female	
	Number	Percentage	Number	Percentage
Accredited MSW	66	51.6	62	48.4
Candidacy MSW	11	52.4	10	47.6
Accredited BSW	158	38.9	248	61.1
Candidacy BSW	11	36.7	19	63.3
Total	246	42.1	339	57.9

authority exists to have an impact on education decisions. Therefore, within the entire spectrum of human categories in social work education including students, faculty, and administrators, women are a distinct majority. Without question, social work education is a feminine enterprise throughout.

Social work education has enunciated and has been guided throughout the educational process by very specific policies that proclaim the value of racial, ethnic, and cultural diversity. Since the 1960s it has rigorously followed the principles of affirmative action in the recruitment of students and the employment of faculty. Programs at both the BSW and MSW levels must infuse content about cultural diversity throughout the curriculum and they face loss of accreditation if they are found lacking in this regard. The area of cultural diversity is rigorously examined at all stages of the accreditation process. Social work students must not only acquire knowledge about minority groups but demonstrate competence in working with persons from culturally diverse populations as a requirement for their degrees.

Given the official commitment and the associated effort that has been devoted to cultural diversity issues in social work education, it might be expected that the field's record in recruiting minority students and faculty would be exemplary. Certainly students and faculty from relevant minority groups should be present in excess of their presence in the population at large. In some cases they are and in some they are not, as the data in Table 5.11 show (U.S. Bureau of the Census, 1997).

The students and faculty that are in social work education beyond their proportion in the total population are white persons, African Americans, and Native Americans. Those present below their percentage in the total population are Chicano/Mexican Americans and Asian Americans. There are no ready explanations for the differences, although it can be reasoned that Asian Americans have a high level of achievement in secondary education and might be attracted to hard science fields rather than social work. It could be expected that Chicano/Mexican Americans might be drawn to social work in larger numbers in the coming decades. With the past emphasis on recruitment of minority students and faculty in social work education the record in this regard cannot be viewed as a successful achievement.

TABLE 5.11. Percentage of Minority Faculty and Students in Social Work Education

Category	Total U.S. Population	BSW Students	MSW Students	Faculty Both Levels
White	72.2	68.0	73.7	77.0
African American	12.1	18.5	12.8	13.9
Native American	0.7	1.4	0.9	0.9
Chicano/Mexican American	11.3	4.3	3.9	2.6
Asian American	3.6	2.2	3.1	2.5
Others	0.1	5.6	5.6	3.1
Total	100.0	100.0	100.0	100.0

CHALLENGES AND OPPORTUNITIES

In spite of the demonstrable strengths exhibited by social work education at both levels, a number of challenges face us at the dawn of the coming century. If these are directly confronted in a spirit of fairness and objectivity by faculty, students, administrators, and professional practitioners they will provide an opportunity for social work education to advance to the next level of relevance and productivity. This chapter has examined the challenges and the authors suggest a series of recommendations for action that are summarily listed below. The manner in which they are dealt with will be an indicator of the potential to educate social workers for a future that remains unknown.

1. The Council on Social Work Education needs to expand its focus beyond intraorganizational maintenance efforts and the accreditation function for individual programs. Priority should be placed on analyzing and determining the need for professionally trained social workers region by region. Following this, programs should be established or continued based on actual need rather than idiosyncratic institutional whims. The first step in this process should be to require all accredited programs to provide evidence that a documented regional need exists for their graduates.

2. Social work education lacks an organizing theory or metanarrative, or system of coherent theories, to provide logical support for its curricular directions. The person-in-environment professional identity

is conceptually broad in the extreme. When this is paired with the perspective of postmodernism, the world of theory adopted by programs becomes bereft of boundaries. Seventy years after the Milford Conference it appears necessary to convene a similar effort to critically review the central purpose of social work education and the conceptual and theoretical foundation upon which it should rest.

3. The Council on Social Work Education maintains minimal standards to which programs must adhere to achieve accreditation. Abundant evidence shows that extreme variation exists among programs that have met the minimal criteria. Interprogram comparative research studies are needed to clearly identify the variable features that are significant to the educational process which are not among the current standards in use.

4. Slavish adherence to the belief that graduate programs should have complete freedom to establish any concentration they wish has led to an excessively broad curriculum. Many concentrations are poorly designed, lack a coherent logic, do not build on relevant theories, are unable to specify expected educational outcomes, and are bereft of content directly related to the concentration. The Council on Social Work Education abandons its responsibility by not providing more stringent guidelines for concentrations that logically flow from the central purpose of social work practice. Accreditation standards must be revised to remedy this problem.

5. Work needs to be done to equalize the fiscal and human resources between undergraduate and graduate social work education programs. This is a symptom of the long-standing tension and competitiveness between the two program levels, and the new century provides the symbolic impetus and opportunity to work toward remedying the disproportionality in these resources.

6. The objectives for BSW students to master generalist knowledge and skills involves a scope of content to be learned that is excessive for the time they spend in the program. Consideration should be given to reexamining the focus of the two program levels—BSW generalist and MSW concentration—to determine if they should be reversed. The decision to produce BSW generalists and MSW specialists was a political decision more than a pedagogical one, and in the climate of century-end change could be revisited.

Chapter 6

Tough Medicine:
What Needs to Be Done

It is clear from the research that most social workers are not involved in knowledge production. The Task Force on Social Work Research (1991) presents some of the most telling evidence concerning this issue. The task force reported that since 1985 fewer than 900 persons had published research in the field, which numbers over 400,000 practitioners. This means that social work depends on only a small cadre of researchers. We also know that social work journals have less impact than journals in related fields. Also, what is published in the area of research articles is often based on rudimentary statistical techniques. Given this state of affairs, it will be difficult for the field of social work to develop a sophisticated theoretical base grounded in rigorous social scientific findings.

In this chapter a number of areas will be developed that will suggest solutions to the problems that confront the field of social work. Specifically, discussion focuses on the need for social workers to ground their knowledge and theory development in epistemologies that stress scientific practice. It will be argued that social work faculty should teach scientific practice; not to do so is simply unethical. It is also suggested that social workers in academic settings must behave like academics in other fields. The importance of grounding curriculum development in empirically based findings is discussed. Finally, it is argued that standards used to select editorial board members must be raised. Journals play a critical role in the development of a profession or discipline. They create a record of how a field meets one of the core requirements of being a profession: possession of a body of knowledge. Since many social work editorial board members often lack publication records and are rarely cited by others, a sound knowledge base is unlikely to emerge from the social work literature.

TOWARD A SCIENTIFIC SOCIAL WORK

In the face of higher education's escalating standards for scholarship, social work faculty are experiencing increased pressure to produce scholarly publications. Social work faculty members who resist this basic requirement are often greatly disappointed when they apply for tenure or promotion. As Euster and Weinbach (1986) note:

> A social work faculty member may emerge from department, school, or college deliberations with strongly endorsed recommendations for tenure and/or promotion and yet become bitterly disappointed where, at other levels of review, he/she may be judged as lacking in achievements expected of an academician. (p. 79)

The denial of tenure or promotion of social work faculty due to the lack of emphasis on scholarship has been well documented. Dinerman (1981) found in her national research on undergraduate and graduate social work programs that many undergraduate programs are staffed by large numbers of nontenured faculty, especially if those faculty lack the usual academic criteria of publications and doctoral degrees. Dinerman suggests that the lack of tenured social work faculty raises concerns of program stability. Furthermore, such programs may face disparagement by academic colleagues who participate in resource allocation and tenure/promotion decisions.

Even though the tradition among social work faculty appears to place secondary emphasis on scholarship, university administrators and social work deans and directors often appear to highly value scholarship as a critical factor for tenure and promotion (Euster and Weinbach, 1986). These findings tend to support Centra's (1979) contention that with fewer faculty members being awarded tenure and promotion, scholarly production becomes more critical. Centra (1979) states:

Research and scholarship, as well as teaching performance, are receiving close scrutiny, focusing in particular on the quality and impact of an individual's work. (p. 119)

In other words, the tradition among social work faculty of stressing practice and service over scholarship is inconsistent with today's academic realities. Social workers within an academic environment must behave and produce at the same levels of scholarship as expected of academics in other fields. What follows is a strategy designed to help social work faculty increase their scholarly productivity.

SCIENTIFIC PRACTICE

Accountability is the buzzword of the 1990s. Within clinical settings, clients often demand proof that the goals of their treatment are being achieved. Funding agencies of social programs are placing similar pressures on agency personnel. This trend can be partially traced to the Health Research Group, one of Ralph Nader's public citizen organizations (Adam and Orgel, 1975).

In the 1980s, the emphasis on accountability emerged in national policy aimed at improving the human services. For example, PL 96-272 (1980), titled the Adoption Assistance and Child Welfare Act, explicitly states that practitioners must have a case plan with clear goals and objectives for every child in placement. The objectives of the case plan must be measurable and time bound. In other words, accountability through empirical validation of services is now national policy for children receiving foster care services.

The demands for accountability from managed care vendors and government agencies are increasing (Sheafor, Hurejsi, and Hurejsi, 1988). Even among clients, the demand for accountability is increasing. The dissatisfaction of clients with treatment outcome has been translated into an increase in malpractice lawsuits. This trend is supported by the rising cost of malpractice insurance as well as courts ruling in favor of clients in an increasing number of lawsuits (Pardeck, 1996).

Even though traditionalists in the social work profession claim clients become upset by systematic evaluation of treatment procedures, the research suggests such is not the case. Campbell (1988) reports that clients often appreciate systematic evaluation grounded in science and not simply the opinions of practitioners.

The demands for accountability provide the social work practitioner-educator with a wealth of opportunities to begin meeting the expectations of scholarship within the academic environment. Through scientific practice, social work educators can achieve not only accountability in practice but also meet the demand for scholarship within the academic community.

Scientific practice, sometimes referred to as "data-guided practice" or "practice research" (Thomas, 1977; Bloom, 1978; Pardeck and Murphy, 1986; Connaway and Gentry, 1988), has led many human services professionals to define the human services as a scientific discipline.

Social workers within the academic setting can meet the emerging emphasis on scholarship by using scientific practice as a means to publication. Briar (1979, pp. 132-133) offers an approach to scientific practice that should be taught as part of social work practice. This approach includes the following steps:

1. Use only methods of intervention known to have empirical validations
2. Continuously evaluate treatment outcome
3. Participate in the testing and reporting of effective practice techniques
4. Use untested practice methods with caution and only with adequate control and evaluation of treatment outcome
5. Communicate the results of evaluation to other professionals

Conducting research in practice is clearly a mandate of the profession. For example, the Council on Social Work Education (1994) now calls for social work educators to understand and appreciate the necessity of the scientific approach to knowledge building and practice, including the scientific evaluation of practice. The recently revised National Association of Social Workers Code of Ethics (NASW, 1996) clearly concludes that scholarship and research are critical to practice and that practitioners must be guided by the conventions of scholarly inquiry.

Many indicators in the field of social work suggest that practice and research should be merged. Indeed, the practitioner-educator in an academic setting should be committed to the production of scholarship not only because it is critical for professional development, but because scientific inquiry is an essential part of practice, according to the Council on Social Work Education and the National Association of Social Workers Code of Ethics. Social work educators have not only the professional obligation to do research, but also to disseminate their findings through professional journals and other available means of informing their colleagues. The outcome of such a strategy will help faculty join the broader academic community in both attitude and behavior. Furthermore, the quality of teaching will be improved because the knowledge and skills presented in the classroom will be based on scientific practice. The most important outcome will be that social work graduates at all levels will be more effective, accountable, and credible practitioners.

AXIOMS OF SCIENTIFIC PRACTICE

An axiom is a principle assumption accepted as self-evidently true (Siporin, 1975). The following eight axioms offer a grounding for scientific practice. They have been developed by Hudson (1984, pp. 185-205) as a set of principles that should guide social work practice as well as theory and knowledge development. These axioms move the social work educator toward objectivism and into the world where problems are assessed, measured, and treated in a scientific fashion:

- *Axiom 1:* If instruments are to have any practice utility they must have two fundamental characteristics: they must be valid, and they must be reliable.

  The importance of this axiom is that regardless of the type of clinical instruments used, it is imperative that they have established reliability and validity.
- *Axiom 2:* For instruments to have maximum utility for social workers, they must be short and easy to administer, understand, score, and interpret.

Often, clinical instruments used in the behavioral or social sciences are long and complicated. Many are difficult to interpret, score, or administer, and some are so technical that only a relatively small number of persons specializing in psychometrics can successfully employ them in practice. Thus, social work practitioners and educators must have instruments available that are easy to score and interpret. Countless scientific instrument are available for practice that meet the criteria of Axiom 2 (Pardeck and Murphy, 1986).

• *Axiom 3:* There are only two ways to determine whether clients have problems: watch them, or ask them.

This axiom means that the practitioner can decide, on the basis of direct observation, whether a client has a problem in some area of social functioning or can simply ask the client to report whether such a problem exists.

• *Axiom 4:* There are only four ways of measuring a client's problem: in terms of its switch, frequency, magnitude, or duration.

If a problem is either present or absent this is referred to as a switch. This is obviously a somewhat crude type of measurement; however, it still has value. Frequency refers to how often the problem occurs. Magnitude measures the degree of presence or absence of a problem. For example, on a scale from 0 to 8, how serious is the depression the client feels? Zero may be coded as no depression present and 8 as serious depression. Finally, duration is simply the length of time a problem has been present.

• *Axiom 5:* If you cannot measure a client's problem it does not exist.

• *Axiom 6:* If you cannot measure a client's problem you cannot treat it.

• *Axiom 7:* If you cannot measure an intervention it does not exist.

• *Axiom 8:* If you cannot measure an intervention you cannot administer it.

The power of the above axioms is that they point to the need to use measurement concepts to formulate and implement treatment. This strategy can lead to the development of scientifically sound knowledge development that social work educators can offer to students in the classroom. The axioms also identify direct linkage between theory and how one can ground theory in measurement.

Most important, they offer a strategy for practitioners and educators to behave and think more scientifically.

Scientific practice offers a sound strategy for social work faculty to translate practice intervention into scholarship. Scientific practice presents an approach for assessing and measuring intervention which can result in a knowledge base that practitioners can use for intervention and one that educators can offer students in the classroom. Speculation and philosophizing about treatment effectiveness become unnecessary because practice intervention is empirically grounded.

Social work educators can be extremely creative in using scientific practice as a research tool. For example, at the macro level of practice, agency and community needs can be measured through a systematic needs assessment design. At the micro level of practice, assessment of client functioning can be more precise through the numerous clinical instruments now available to practice. Practice effectiveness can also be measured through the single-subject design. The single-subject design has been found to be a very useful research strategy that allows practitioners to measure the occurrence of a problem and develop a means for monitoring clinical changes. Likewise, content analysis can be an extremely powerful research design for understanding treatment effectiveness (Pardeck and Pardeck, 1987). Social work educators have numerous methodologies available for conducting scientific research in the community. The findings from this research offer countless opportunities for scholarly publication.

A SCIENTIFICALLY BASED THEORY OF SOCIAL WORK PRACTICE

Social work faculty have an ethical obligation to teach intervention techniques that work. Thyer (1997) concludes that not using scientifically sound techniques for practice intervention is a violation of the ethical standards of the profession. Furthermore, if social work faculty are teaching intervention approaches that do not work, they are not meeting their ethical obligations to students. Van Houten and colleagues (1988) conclude the following about the importance of teaching scientifically sound intervention strategies:

An individual has a right to the most effective treatment procedures available. In turn, [clinicians] have an obligation to use only those techniques that have been demonstrated by researchers to be effective, to acquaint consumers and the public with the advantages and disadvantages of these techniques, and to search continuously for the most optimal means of changing behavior. (p. 113)

For a variety of reasons, social workers in all practice settings, including academic, do not keep abreast of recent developments in effective psychosocial interventions (Thyer, 1997). If we assume there is a finite number of different client problems for which professional attention is warranted, each new empirical advance in clinical research fills in the map leading toward more effective treatments. Presently, we do have two theories of intervention that offer social workers scientifically sound interventions; behavioral intervention and cognitive therapeutic intervention. The following briefly reviews each theory, including their scientific basis. It will be argued that these theories should be the grounding for practice courses because they provide students with intervention strategies based in scientific practice.

Behavioral Intervention

A number of theorists are associated with behavior theory (e.g., Ivan Pavlov and John B. Watson). However, B. F. Skinner (1953) is the theorist who has had the greatest influence on this orientation to assessment and intervention. Skinner did not develop new principles of behaviorism; instead he translated the theories and ideas of other behaviorists into an applied and useful therapeutic technology. His methods are widely used in psychology, counseling, and psychiatry—they should also be a dominant intervention approach in social work (Pardeck, 1996).

From a behavioral perspective, individuals are viewed as biological entities that respond to the events which happen to them. People are seen as largely products of their environment. In other words, individuals are responders to their environments, and these environments shape both functional and dysfunctional behavior (Pardeck, 1996).

From an intervention point of view, social workers using behavioral techniques are grounded in a stimulus-response paradigm. Clients are seen as entities that respond in a predictable fashion to any given stimulus according to what they have learned through previous life experience. Humans react in essentially the same fashion as infrahumans to stimuli, except that these responses are more organized and complex (Pardeck, 1996).

Skinner viewed people as programmed with a repertoire of responses that are repeated over and over. In essence, people learn specific responses that satisfy environmental conditions. What this means is that individual behavior is very predictable; it also becomes obvious that environmental conditions play a central role in determining behavior. Given this principle, the role of the social worker is one of helping clients to unlearn dysfunctional behaviors and replace these with new behaviors. A number of scientifically based principles have been identified that help clients unlearn behaviors that create problems. Behavioral intervention is a reeducation or relearning process. Positive behaviors are reinforced, and dysfunctional behaviors are extinguished. Through reinforcement principles, the client learns functional behavior and unlearns dysfunctional behavior (Pardeck, 1996)

Assessment through behavioral analysis follows these basic steps: (a) identify the presenting problem, (b) determine the cause of the problem, and (c) select a solution. The solution, or intervention, will involve positive reinforcement of functional behaviors and the elimination of undesired behaviors. Some behavioral problems are typically viewed as rooted in antecedents and consequences; these processes thus become the focus of intervention. What is powerful about this approach to assessment is that it works and it is grounded in science (Pardeck, 1996).

A goal of behavior intervention is to help the client learn strategies for coping. From a philosophical viewpoint, all behavior can be changed—the problem is finding the appropriate positive or negative stimuli to accomplish this goal. Numerous techniques are available to reduce or eliminate anxiety, obsessive behaviors, phobias, depression, and other problematic behaviors (Krumboltz, 1966; Krumboltz and Hosford, 1967). These researchers have identified four main categories for organizing goals of behavioral intervention:

1. Alerting the client to maladaptive behavior.
2. Teaching the decision-making process.
3. Preventing problems.
4. Teaching new behaviors and skills.

Once a problem is identified, the clinician can use a variety of counseling techniques to help a client modify behavior to solve a presenting problem. A major goal of behavioral intervention is to teach clients self-management skills they can apply to various life situations. Through this approach clients learn to become their own behavioral modification experts (Pardeck, 1996).

Behaviorists are sensitive to what is referred to as the intraself; however, since this intraself cannot be seen directly, they prefer to work with observable results of these internal psychological processes. The guiding principle behind this position is that if the symptoms can be changed (overt behavior), the internal psychological causes are of secondary importance. In other words, what is critical to the behaviorist is changing those activities that contribute to problems, and not necessarily their causes (Pardeck, 1996).

A number of techniques can be employed when using behavioral intervention. These include contingency contracting, self-management, shaping, biofeedback, and modeling. The following is an example of contingency contracting, which involves five steps:

1. Identify the problem.
2. Collect baseline data to understand events associated with the problem.
3. Set goals to solve the problem.
4. Select techniques for obtaining the goals.
5. If goals are not reached, establish new behavioral change strategies.

The process is clearly grounded in science; furthermore, a single-subject methodology neatly fits this approach. A single-subject methodology should be a core technology of social work practice (Pardeck, 1996).

Self-management is a strategy that helps clients learn how to take control of their lives. The major difference between self-management and other behavioral approaches is that the client assumes responsibility for changing behavior. The intervention process includes the following steps:

1. Define the problem in behavioral terms.
2. Collect data on the problem.
3. Introduce a treatment plan based on behavioral principles.
4. Evaluate the plan.
5. If the plan is not working, change it.

Presently, numerous self-management books and manuals are available to help clients change problem behaviors (Pardeck, 1994).

Shaping is an operant technique to induce new behaviors by reinforcing ones that approximate the desired behavior. Through this process the client gradually achieves the desired behavior. The technique involves (a) looking, (b) waiting, and (c) reinforcing. In other words, the practitioner waits for the client to exhibit positive behavior, then reinforces this behavior. Through the shaping process the client gradually develops appropriate behaviors (Pardeck, 1996).

Modeling is another scientifically sound technique for shaping behavior. This technique includes using books, videotapes, and other resources to teach functional behaviors. The practitioner may also serve as a model (Pardeck, 1996). A goal of modeling is to help the client gain awareness of how his or her behavior is controlled and shaped by the environment. The following steps are an example of how videotaping can be used through modeling:

1. The client identifies behaviors that he or she wishes to change.
2. Through videotaping, the practitioner gathers baseline data associated with the undesirable behavior.
3. The practitioner offers other models through videotape that illustrate more desirable behavior.
4. The client practices these new positive behaviors while being videotaped and gradually learns the desired behaviors. Exposure to positive models has been effective regardless of whether the model or the observer receives visible reinforcement.

The research literature offers numerous techniques that practitioners can use for conducting behavioral intervention (e.g., Pardeck, 1994). Furthermore, the research literature clearly shows that behavioral approaches are effective. Behaviorist theorists were also the first to mount a significant attack on psychodynamic models that were widely used prior to the development of behavior theory. Many of these models continue to dominate social work practice even though they have limited scientific support. Finally, social work faculty should teach behavioral interventions because they are scientifically sound and they allow practitioners to document effectiveness in practice (Pardeck, 1996).

Cognitive Therapeutic Intervention

The focus of cognitive therapy is on psychological disturbances caused by aberrations in thinking. The role of the therapist is to help clients develop psychological skills to correct this condition. These skills include labeling and interpreting negative psychological disturbances and ultimately correcting these conditions through intervention (Pardeck, 1996).

Cognitive therapy demands that clients have the capacity for introspection and reflection. These processes enable clients to increase self-awareness and the ability to substitute accurate judgments for inaccurate judgments. Not all clients have the cognitive or intellectual capacity to engage in this form of intervention (Pardeck, 1996).

A number of therapists represent the cognitive therapeutic approach, including Beck (1976), Glasser (1969), and Ellis (1997)— Ellis is clearly the leading figure in the field of cognitive therapy.

Ellis views human beings as largely irrational and believes they need to be taught rational approaches for dealing with problems. Humans think crookedly about their desires and preferences, thus resulting in anger, anxiety, depression, and self-pity. Unfortunately, irrational thinking leads to self-hate, which may lead to self-destructive behavior and eventually to hatred of others (Pardeck, 1996).

Thompson and Rudolph (1992) list a number of irrational beliefs that cause people trouble, based on the work of Ellis:

1. It is a necessity for me to be loved by everyone in whatever I attempt to do.
2. People should be thoroughly competent and adequate in all possible respects.
3. Certain individuals are wicked and they should be punished because of this.
4. It is terrible when things are not going well for me.
5. Unhappiness is externally caused; people have little or no ability to control sorrow or rid themselves of their negative thoughts and feelings.
6. If something is dangerous, one must be totally occupied with this danger.

The goal of rational-emotive therapy is to teach people to think and behave in a more functional fashion. Furthermore, people must take responsibility for the self, including their own logical thinking and the behaviors that result from their thinking. By teaching clients to reflect on their thinking, the consequences resulting from that thinking can be corrected. Finally, the critical point about cognitive therapy intervention is that it is scientifically sound and it works. Cognitive techniques should be a dominant therapeutic method taught by social work faculty (Pardeck, 1996).

Behavioral and cognitive interventions have been shown to be highly effective and grounded in science. A behavioral approach is particularly consistent with social work practice because of its emphasis on the importance of the environment in shaping client behavior, a view clearly aligned with a traditional social work perspective (Pardeck, 1996).

Cognitive therapeutic intervention can also be a useful approach supporting social work practice because it helps clients deal more effectively with environmental constraints. Cognitive techniques can be effective in helping clients improve their interaction with their social environments. For example, parents who are having interpersonal problems with a child who is not living up to their expectations must be taught rational approaches to dealing with their youngsters. Parents who demand perfection are probably approaching their children from an irrational perspective. This irrationality creates a process of transaction between parents and child that may result in dysfunctional behavior. Countless problems can be corrected if cognitive techniques are used to help clients change their interaction with the various systems composing their social environments (Pardeck, 1996).

Psychodynamic approaches, treatment strategies that largely emphasize the intrapsychic in both assessment and intervention, have limited utility for social workers because they are not grounded in science. As suggested earlier by Thyer (1997), social work faculty teaching psychodynamic techniques may well be behaving unethically because these techniques have limited scientific support. Those who teach scientifically based theories of intervention such as behavior and cognitive approaches are acting ethically (Pardeck, 1996).

BEHAVING LIKE OTHER ACADEMICS

One of the unusual aspects of social work education at the doctoral level is the limited number of graduates receiving a doctorate in social work. Many of those who earn the doctorate are of advanced age, which means foreshortened research careers. Future efforts should be made to recruit a larger number of students into the field earlier in their careers—this should help to ensure more years of research productivity.

There is clearly insufficient research and statistical training at the MSW and doctorate levels, both in amount and sophistication. The lack of solid course work in research appears to contribute to the relatively low production rates among doctoral graduates and social work faculty in general. This not only means social work programs have limited standing in the academic community, but also it is difficult to obtain grants from funding agencies. Presently, schools of social work are environments in which federally funded research projects and research assistantships are few in number, prolific researchers are rare, and many graduate-level faculty lack doctoral degrees. A remedy for this problem might be to increase the number of doctoral programs offering social work education and to consider the doctorate in social work as the terminal degree in the field, not the MSW degree. These changes would drive the demand for the social work doctorate; they would also help to ensure that more faculty holding doctorates are hired in schools of social work.

Fraser, Lewis, and Norman (1990) concluded that a continuum of education is needed in social work from the bachelor's level to the doctorate level. The thrust of this continuum should be to integrate statistical and research methodological training across the social work curriculum at all educational levels. A sequence approach would help to eliminate redundancy in programming at different educational levels and would enhance the acquisition of advanced research techniques. It is critical that the research technologies that are taught be current and within the parameters of acceptable science. This for some time has not been the case at the MSW level. For example, Grinnell, Kyte, and Hunter (1979) twenty years ago found that doctorate programs had integrity in the area of research; however, they reported such was not the case for undergraduate and MSW programs:

> In view of the virtual nonexistence of research component in undergraduate social work education—and its dramatic, progressive erosion at the master's level—the study findings provide a measure of welcome relief. While the research component has been moving toward—or has already reached—the "twilight zone" in certain spheres of social work academia, its integrity at the doctoral level would appear to be intact. (p. 383)

Unfortunately limited progress has been made in developing the quality of research training at the MSW level since the 1970s.

Fraser (1994) argues that a "culture of scholarship" must be established at more schools of social work. This will only occur if scholarship is rewarded at meaningful levels. One strategy that would facilitate scholarly productivity is to adjust academic workloads to allow for greater production of scholarship. Innovative strategies for increasing production are offered by a number of writers. Berger (1990) presents a program in one school of social work that helps faculty increase publication rates.

Schilling, Schinke, and Gilchrist (1985) examine ways researchers can publish their findings that offer the greatest interest to practitioners. Pardeck (1991) presents a program for using scientifically based practice as an approach for increasing scholarly activity among social work educators.

Finally, the most important change that must occur is to insist that promotion and tenure criteria not only include a solid record of teaching and service but also scholarship. The findings are similar on the lack of scholarly production at all academic levels of social work education. Consistently, a majority of all studies have concluded that most social work faculty are not productive in the area of scholarship. Even among faculties of the schools of social work where scholarly production is a major occupational expectation, the percentage of faculty who report giving papers at conferences, having articles published in professional and academic journals, and writing books and book chapters is very low. In 1989, as an example, data collected by the Council on Social Work Education showed that total scholarly productivity for faculty in member institutions equaled less than one journal article for every two faculty, and about one book and one book chapter for every six faculty (Spaulding, 1991). Green, Hutchinson, and Sar (1992), in a recent study of more than 1,700 social work doctoral graduates, found that active participation in scholarly activities was the exception, rather than the rule, among those receiving the doctorate. Almost half of the graduates had not published a single article in a social work journal over their entire careers. A third had not made a minimum of one presentation at a social work conference since receiving their doctorate and more than half had not written a book chapter. This research did in fact, however, find that a small number of scholars within the field produced the majority of the articles published in social work journals.

As long as schools of social work grant tenure and promotion on the basis of nontraditional academic standards—which has seemingly been the case—a "culture of scholarship" will not emerge. In essence, faculty members who suggest that they are too busy to produce scholarship because of teaching and service commitments should not be granted tenure or promotion.

IMPROVING SOCIAL WORK EDITORIAL BOARDS

The findings concerning social work editorial boards show convincing evidence that many manuscript reviewers do not have records of scholarly production. These findings suggest changes should be made in how manuscript reviewers are selected. Presently the selection process for editorial board appointment does not appear to be based on the traditional standards used in other disciplines such as psychology and sociology (Lindsey, 1976). These traditional standards include a record of publication that has resulted in a meaningful contribution to a given field. To correct this condition a number of strategies should be implemented (Pardeck, 1994).

It may be time for social work journals to use the same kind of strategies implemented in hiring faculty members. When social work programs seek new faculty members they attempt to identify those who have the talent and competence to perform the tasks required for positions that need to be filled. This is accomplished through making those positions known to the profession, which then allows those who feel they qualify to apply. A similar approach should be used for the selection of editorial board members. Presently, the approach used to appoint individuals to social work editorial boards is surrounded in mystery. The only criterion that is apparently not used for a significant number of appointments is a record of research and scholarly publication (Pardeck, 1996).

Finally, the profession of social work needs a greater commitment to research and scholarship; social work educators must lead this reform. Such critical reform within the academic community will ultimately push the intellectual quality of the profession to new levels. The quality of social work journals will only improve if those who determine what new information and knowledge will appear in them, which is thus presumably consumed by practitioners, have the competence to fulfill this function. Central to this competence is a scholarly record of distinction and achievement as documented by publication in peer-reviewed journals, and evidence that their work is being used by other scholars as measured by citations of their work. Since the 1970s, many of those who have served on social work editorial boards do not have a record of scholarly production. The field of social work will not develop a strong knowledge base until manuscript reviewers are appointed to social work editorial boards based on their distinction and achievements made through the publication process—editorial board appointment is presently based on unknown criteria that clearly do not include scholarly achievement.

SUMMARY AND CONCLUSION

In this chapter a number of strategies have been presented for moving the field of social work forward. Most of these strategies can be easily achieved if there were only an openness to the basic canons of science for testing and building knowledge.

Specifically, scientific practice should be used as the approach to building new knowledge in the field. Using pseudoscience as a basis for knowledge development will only mean that social workers will continue to use social interventions that have no scientific validity. Academics in schools of social work must be the leaders in ensuring that students and practitioners understand the importance of building knowledge through scientific rigor.

It has also been suggested that social work journals must ensure that editorial board appointment is based on merit as reflected through sound scholarly productivity. Journals are one of the most important mediums through which a knowledge base is built in all disciplines and professions.

Finally, Carl Sagan's (1997) work, *The Demon-Haunted World: Science As a Candle in the Dark,* offers an excellent analysis concerning knowledge building in all professional or academic fields. Sagan suggests that much of what people believe is based on myth and pseudoscience. Unfortunately, much of the knowledge base in social work also suffers from these problems. Social workers must begin to view the social world though the eyes of the skeptic—for this is what science is about. For example, when a colleague claims that his or her twenty years of practice experience has resulted in a valid knowledge base that students must be exposed to—the response should be that he or she must prove the validity of his or her practice experience through scientific rigor before it becomes valid knowledge. Until this is done, practice experience is nothing more than knowledge based on myth and belief.

This kind of skepticism is rare in the field of social work. Scientists reject mystic revelation, a category under which one can easily classify practice experience, as a valid source of knowledge guiding practice; particularly as a source for knowledge taught in the classroom. Science opens new paths of thought and approaches. The field of social work clearly suffers by not using science as a tool for opening new doors that may well lead to important discoveries. Sagan's (1997) work concerning the importance of science for understanding the world is summarized in the following quote. In a certain sense, it is a precise summary of the thinking and behavior that the field of social work needs to move forward:

> The scientific way of thinking is at once imaginative and disciplined. This is central to its success. Science invites us to let the facts in, even when they don't conform to our preconceptions. It counsels us to carry alternative hypotheses in our heads and see which best fit the facts. It urges on us a delicate balance between no-holds-barred openness to new ideas, however heretical, and the most rigorous skeptical scrutiny of everything—new ideas and established wisdom. (p. 27)

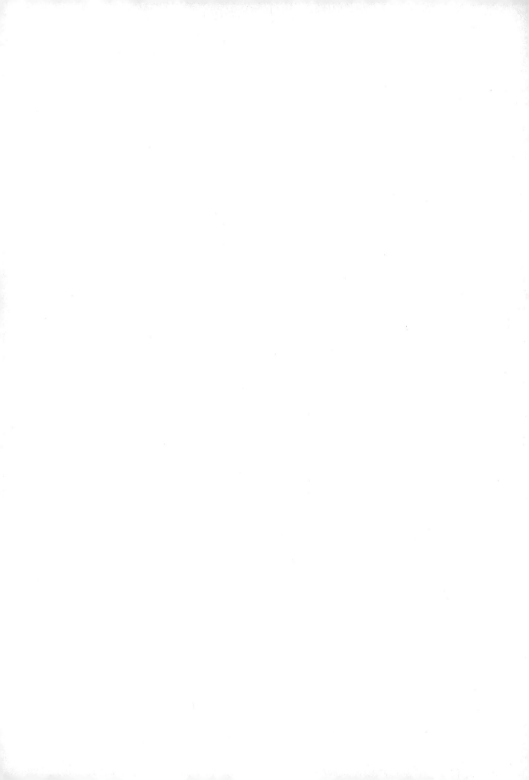

Chapter 7

Critical Issues
for the Twenty-First Century

In some respects, common issues face contemporary social work as it transits from the twentieth to the twenty-first century that are similar to those of a hundred years ago. Both now and then events and discoveries in the scientific, business, educational, and cultural domains were having a major impact on the way people thought and conducted their daily lives. At both times changes were occurring with profound consequences for the following decades and that left their mark on the professions. The country's population makeup and its characteristics a hundred years ago underwent rapid changes. During the years 1880 to 1915 approximately 21 million immigrants came to the United States and the birthrate of the native population was on the rise. These millions from both outside and inside the country worked hard to adapt to a nation on the move. The strangers to the new culture were striving to create new communities and assimilate themselves into the ways of the country of their choice. The challenges facing these new citizens were similar to those that face the ethnic and cultural minorities of the present time. The earlier immigrants became part of a dynamic of an increasing industrial structure that was flexing its muscles, resulting in a rapidly changing social and economic landscape. At the dawn of the twentieth century education, the political scene, the arts, and the cultural climate were entering a period of modernity and progressiveness. Perhaps the development with the most impact and greatest consequences at the time was the rise of science, which provided an underlying foundation for education, industry, and the professions. The modern scientific achievements of the early 1900s had an impact on a par with the computer revolution, the hypertechnological developments, and the social and moral revolution of the past two decades. It was during the period of social progress and scientific modernity of the late nineteenth and early twentieth centuries that social work was in an embryonic stage and in the process of creating itself. Now, a century later, social work, having passed through a variety of developmental phases, is facing conditions requiring it to reinvent itself. Even though the changes now occurring in the country are postindustrial and postmodern in nature, their impact on society is no less dramatic than those of a century ago. The late twentieth-century changes constitute a context for the major challenges and opportunities facing social work that have been explored and examined in this book.

The previous chapters have presented challenges variously described under the headings of theory, grand narrative, paradigm, or basic foundational logic. These challenges face both the field of practice and education and they raise basic concerns about the survival of the profession. After social work had moved through its early developmental years, there emerged what might be called a series of professional superegos or theoretical perspectives that provided a lens for viewing and understanding social reality. They provided an organizing framework by which individual and social problems could be categorized, diagnosed, and treated. These perspectives also created a shared culture and value system that provided a unifying bond among social workers as well as a guide for their professional actions. These perspectives included the psychoanalytic, systems, ecological, behavioral, and role theory as well as a few others of lesser stature. It is not possible to concretely state when each perspective was developed and then subsequently declined, but roughly the sixty years from 1925 through 1985 comprise their viable span of greatest impact. In recent years they have broken up due to splintered cultural identities, massive migrations, scientific developments, the revolution in computer hypertechnologies, and unprecedented social and cultural upheavals. In some sense social work has become similar to what in research is called a dependent variable. It does not itself function as an influence for other variables but is influenced by them. There have arisen numerous fields of practice; populations to be served; technologies to be used; and a hierarchy of human system levels to be considered. Social workers find themselves responding to and dependent on this constellation of forces, and they function according to their demands. They have no grand narrative or economical set of theories to guide their work, resulting in a lack of autonomous practice. In a word, they have become a commodity. The result for social work has been the elimination of a set of organizing theories to guide research, education, and practice and their replacement by numerous perspectives emerging from geographic location or organizational auspices. These theoretical fads lack the power to bind the profession together, resulting in an array of interest groups with short-lived impact. Each field of practice appears to have its own preferred fad that separates it from other fields. Fads also have appeal in social work education, where curricula exhibit extreme variation from program to program, particularly in regard to graduate concentrations. The solution is not readily evident and answers cannot be pursued until the problem is recognized throughout the profession. At this time, such recognition does not exist and it will not as long as the market opportunities for social workers remain strong and enrollment in education programs continues to increase. It is likely that social work will only face this issue head-on after a market or educational crisis appears.

In the first half of the century social work passionately pursued an identity that would permit it to lay claim to being a scientifically based profession. Within the system of helping professions, particularly with psychiatry and psychology, it negotiated energetically to be accepted at their level. Within higher education it strove mightily to be classified along with other long-standing professions as an autonomous and independent field. In both respects, but in varying degrees, it achieved these aspirations to be a science-based profession deserving a specific place as a university-based educational program. As social work abandons empirically based science, its knowledge base is diluted and it borrows heavily from other social and psychological disciplines. In addition, serious questions have been raised about the quality of manuscript reviews of social work journals, which function as the main mechanism whereby information is disseminated to practitioners. In earlier times social work was able to lay sole claim to fields of practice such as child welfare. It no longer can do that, but finds itself a participant along with other social professions in an increasingly wide range of practice fields.

The entire world is currently caught up in the ever-increasing and seemingly never-ending appearance of computer-based hypertechnology and the interconnected field of associated developments that have created a new cyberspace environment. Without question the field of hypertechnology is totally market driven and based on profit motives. It is also impersonal in the extreme and operates outside the social and psychological dynamics of meaningful human experience. The past two decades have witnessed the adoption within social work of most of the hypertechnological advances without a reasoned examination of their consequences. We have argued that long-standing and cherished attributes of social work may have been negatively impacted by the computer revolution. They have diminished social work's value perspectives and caused the loss of personal freedom, the centralization of power among the anointed few, and most important, the diminution of social interaction. Clearly the abundance of information available to researchers in computerized databases has moved the focus away from studying the day-to-day human problems of client groups toward issues prompted by the existence of the data itself. Perhaps more trivial research is underway using office-available data instead of in situ studies with individuals, families, and communities that have the objective of solving real-life problems.

In addition to the challenges of a scientific and theoretical nature, the entire spectrum of social work education seems to be moving toward curricular chaos and parochialism. Two problems stand out. The first is the inappropriateness and mismatch of official educational focus at the baccalaureate (BSW) and master's (MSW) levels. At the first level (BSW), where the students have less academic experience, the most comprehensive and wide-ranging array of content is presented. At the second level (MSW), where the students have the most academic experience, the most specialized content is presented. Many experts argue that this order should be reversed. The second problem is at the graduate (MSW) level, where all the CSWE-accredited programs, which number over 125, have the absolute freedom to select any specialized concentration they wish. A CSWE policy, widely ignored, states that these concentrations must rest on a body of theory and a confirmed knowledge base. A few do, but most do not. Those with concentrations in health, for example, rest on a body of empirically generated knowledge that supports their curricular logic. Other concentrations are organized around practice roles, population groups, problem manifestations, or contemporary interests that lack supporting theory or knowledge. Concentrations across programs have nothing to logically or epistemologically bind them together. Thus, when people ask the question, "What do social workers do?" they get as many answers as there are practitioners who answer them.

As the twenty-first century begins it is questionable whether social work will remain among the family of major helping professions. It does not unequivocally meet all the major attributes of what constitutes a profession, and it is difficult to assign it to an indisputable niche sanctioned by society. To remain at the level of a major profession is its central challenge as well as its opportunity. This book has presented an analysis of the issues facing social work and a few recommendations for meeting the challenges. Throughout the analysis it is clear that social work may not control its own fate. The forces of hypertechnology, the power of the marketplace that dictates the direction in which professions function, the stifling bureaucracies in which most social workers are employed, the absence of a core organizing grand narrative, and an increasingly directionless educational establishment appear to be negative factors detracting from the control social work has over its destiny. There may be many in the social work profession who take issue and disagree with the analysis that has been provided. It is the opinion of the authors that these issues must be squarely, openly, and honestly faced if social work is to seize the few opportunities that might be available to it at the beginning of the twenty-first century.

The fundamental theme of this book is that social work faces a series of challenges to be met and overcome if it is to move into the coming century as a relevant and viable profession. Prefatory to dealing with the challenges is the establishment within the culture of social work a new spirit and institutional life force. For this spirit to flourish, a number of actions must be taken. One of these actions is the elimination of the domination of dialogue by special interest groups. If open inquiry and exploration of new and novel directions is to take place, all need to have a place at the communication table, not just a few. It is tragic that social work, with its historical commitment to social justice, has in recent years permitted itself to be dominated by a small number of ideological interest groups. It has been noted that those outside these special interest groups are wary about discussing their positions because the communicative climate is so hostile. Social work must also demonstrate the will to resist the private-sector, market-force-driven influence over the provision of services. It cannot, for example, condone and participate in a system of managed care health services driven by the profit motive when it is estimated that about fifty million people are without health insurance and another fifty million are underinsured. Lastly, the phenomenal hypertechnological developments are not a blessing for all. Already there are technological haves and have-nots, and the breach is becoming as serious as the gaps in income. In social work, as enormous amounts of data are generated, stored, and retrieved, the human person and his or her unique needs seem to become secondary to nonhuman information. If, as argued throughout the book, grand narratives are to be produced, they must be ones that have a human face and not ones dominated by machines.

References

Chapter 1

Abbott, A. (1988). *The system of professions.* Chicago: The University of Chicago Press.

Baker, D. and Wilson, M. (1992). An evaluation of the scholarly productivity of doctoral graduates. *Journal of Social Work Education,* 28(2):204-213.

Beverly, S. and Sherraden, M. (1997). Investment in human development as a social development strategy. *Social Development Issues,* 19(1):1-18.

Billups, J. (1990). Toward social development as an organizing concept for social work and related social professions and movements. *Social Development Issues,* 12(3):14-26.

Bisno, H. and Cox, F. (1997). Social work education: Catching up with the present and future. *Journal of Social Work Education,* 33(2):373-387.

CSWE (1992a). *Curriculum policy statement for baccalaureate degree programs in social work education.* Alexandria, VA: Council on Social Work Education.

CSWE (1992b). *Curriculum policy statement for master's degree programs in social work education.* Alexandria, VA: Council on Social Work Education.

CSWE (1994). *Master's evaluative standards and interpretive guidelines.* Alexandria, VA: Council on Social Work Education.

Epstein, W. (1990). Confirmation response bias among social work journals. *Science, Technology, and Human Values,* 15(1):9-38.

Estes, R. (1990). Development under different political and economic systems. *Social Development Issues,* 13(1):5-19.

Flexner, A. (1915). Is social work a profession? *Proceedings of the National Conference of Charities and Corrections.* Chicago: Hildman Printing, pp. 576-590.

Haack, S. (1992). Science "from a feminist perspective." *Philosophy,* 67:5-18.

Hartman, A. (1992). In search of subjugated knowledge. *Social Work,* 37:483-484.

Howard, M. and Lambert, M. (1996). The poverty of social work: Deficient production, dissemination, and utilization of practice-relevant scientific information. In Raffoul, P. and McNeece, C. (Eds.), *Future issues for social work practice* (pp. 279-292). Needham Heights, MA: Allyn and Bacon.

Karger, H. (1994). Toward redefining social development in the global economy: Free markets, privatization, and the development of a welfare state in eastern Europe. *Social Development Issues,* 16(3):32-44.

Meinert, R. (1998). Consequences for professional social work under conditions of postmodernity. *Social Thought,* 18(3):41-54.

Midgley, J. (1990). International social work: Learning from the third world. *Social Work,* 35(4):295-301.

Pardeck, J. (1992). Are social work journal editorial boards competent? Some disquieting data with implications for research on social work practice. *Research on Social Work Practice,* 2(4):487-496.

Pardeck, J. and Meinert, R. (1994). Do social workers have a major impact on social policy? In Karger, H. and Midgley, J. (Eds.), *Controversial issues in social policy* (pp. 93-106). New York: Allyn and Bacon.

Pozatek, E. (1994). The problem of certainty: Clinical social work in the postmodern era. *Social Work,* 39(4):396-403.

Sands, R. and Nuccio, K. (1992). Postmodern feminist theory and social work. *Social Work,* 37(6):489-494.

Tucker, D. (1996). Eclecticism is not a free good: Barriers to knowledge development in social work. *Social Service Review,* 70:400-434.

Weick, A. (1993). Reconstructing social work education. *Journal of Teaching in Social Work,* 8(1/2):11-30.

Wilson, E. (1998). *Consilience: The unity of knowledge.* New York: Alfred A. Knopf, Inc.

Chapter 2

Abramovitz, M. (1986). The privatization of the welfare state: A review. *Social Work,* 31(4):261-262.

Agger, B. (1991). *A critical theory of public life: Knowledge, discourse and politics in an age of decline.* New York: The Falmer Press.

Agger, B. (1995). *Fast capitalism.* Boulder, CO: Westview Press.

Agger, B. (1998). *Critical social theory: An introduction.* Boulder, CO: Westview Press.

Appadurai, A. (1990). Disjuncture and difference in global cultural economy. *Public Culture,* 2(2):10.

Banton, M. (1987). *Radical theories.* Cambridge, UK: Cambridge University Press.

Barker, M. and Hardiker, P. (Eds.). (1981). *Theories of practice in social work.* London: Academic Press.

Baudrillard, J. (1988). *Baudrillard: Selected writings,* M. Poster (Ed.). Stanford, CA: Stanford University Press.

Berman, M. (1982). *All that is solid melts into air: The experience of modernity.* New York: Simon and Schuster.

Booth, D. (1994). *Rethinking social development: Theory, research and practice.* London: Longman.

Brahm, G. and Driscoll, M. (1995). *Prosthetic territories: Politics and hypertechnologies.* Boulder, CO: Westview Press.

Brennan, W. (1973). The practitioner as theoretician. *Journal of Education for Social Work,* 9(1):5-12.

Bryner, G. (1998). *Politics and public morality: The great American welfare reform debate.* New York: W.W. Norton and Company.

Chambon, A. and Irving, A. (Eds.). (1994). *Essays in postmodernism and social work.* Toronto: Canadian Scholars Press.

Chernus, L.A. (1995). Social workers: Fallen angels or mere mortals? An essay review of *Unfaithful angels: How social work has abandoned its mission. Clinical Social Work Journal,* 23(3):375-382.

Collins, B. (1986). Defining feminist social work. *Social Work,* 31(3):214-219.

Conner, S. (1989). *Postmodernist Culture: An introduction to the theories of the contemporary.* Cambridge, MA: Basic Blackwell Inc.

Davis, L. (1985). Female and male voices in social work. *Social Work,* 30(2): 106-113.

Dawkins, R. (1986). *The blind watchmaker: Why the evidence of evolution reveals a universe without design.* New York: W.W. Norton and Company.

Dawkins, R. (1995). God's utility function. *Scientific American,* 273(5):80-85.

Dodgshon, R. (1998). *Society in time and space: A geographical perspective on change.* Cambridge, UK: Cambridge University Press.

Dore, M. (1990). Functional theory: Its history and influence on contemporary social work. *Social Service Review,* 64:358-374.

Drucker, P. (1993). *Post-capitalist society.* New York: HarperCollins.

Epstein, W. (1990). The obligation of intellectuals. *Science, Technology, and Human Values,* 15(1):244-247.

Epstein, W. (1995). Social work in the university. *Journal of Social Work Education,* 31(2):281-291.

Fischer, R. and Karger, H. (1997). *Social work and community in a private world: Getting out in public.* New York: Longman.

Forder, A. (1976). Social work and systems theory. *British Journal of Social Work,* 6(1):24-41.

Foucault, M. (1990). *Knowledge/power.* New York: Pantheon.

Germain, C. and Gitterman, A. (1980). *The life model of social work practice.* New York: Columbia University Press.

Gibbs, W.W. (1995). Seeking the criminal element. *Scientific American,* 272(3): 100-107.

Goffman, E. (1963). *Behavior in public places: Notes on the social organization of gatherings.* New York: The Free Press.

Gomory, T. (1997). Social work and philosophy. In Reisch, M. and Gambrill, E. (Eds.), *Social work in the 21st century* (pp. 300-310). Thousand Oaks, CA: Pine Forge Press.

Gottdiener, M. (1985). *The social production of urban space.* Austin, TX: University of Texas Press.

Greene, R. and Ephross, P. (1991). *Human behavior theory and social work practice.* New York: Aldine De Gruyter.

Greenwood, A. (1992). *Science at the frontier.* Washington, DC: National Academy Press.

Habermas, J. (1987). *Theory of communicative action.* Boston: Beacon Press.

Harvey, D. (1989). *The conditions of postmodernity: An inquiry into the origins of cultural change.* Cambridge, MA: Basil Blackwell.

Hearn, J. (1982). The problem(s) of theory and practice in social work and social work education. *Issues in Social Work Education,* 2(2):95-118.

Heineman, M. (1981). The obsolete scientific imperative in social work research. *Social Service Review,* 55(3):371-397.

Howe, D. (1994). Modernity, post-modernity and social work. *British Journal of Social Work,* 24(5):513-532.

Howe, D. (1995). *An introduction to social work theory.* Aldershot Berks, UK: Wildwood House.

Imre, R. (1984). The nature of knowledge in social work. *Social Work,* 29(1):41-45.

Karger, H. (1986). Science, research, and social work: Who controls the profession? *Social Work,* 28(3):200-205.

Karger, H. and Stoesz, D. (1998). *American social welfare policy: A pluralist approach,* Third edition. New York: Longman.

Kitchin, R. (1998). *Cyberspace: The world in the wires.* New York: John Wiley and Sons.

Kreuger, L. (1997). The end of social work. *Journal of Social Work Education,* 33(1):19-27.

Kreuger, L. (1999). Shallow science. *Research on Social Work Practice,* 9(1):108-110.

Krill, D. (1976). *Existential social work.* New York: Free Press.

Kuhn, T. (1970). *The structure of scientific revolutions.* Chicago: University of Chicago Press.

Lapham, V. (1996). Tough questions posed on genetic tests. *NASW News, Washington DC,* 41(2):5.

Lefebvre, H. (1991). *The production of space.* Cambridge, MA: Blackwell Publishers.

Lindley, D. (1993). *The end of physics: The myth of a unified theory.* New York: HarperCollins.

Lischman, J. (Ed.). (1991). *Handbook of theory for practice teachers in social work.* London: Jessica Kingsley.

Longres, J. (1997). The impact and implications of multiculturalism. In Reisch, M. and Gambrill, E. (Eds.), *Social work in the 21st century* (pp. 39-47). Thousand Oaks, CA: Pine Forge Press.

Manchester, W. (1974). *The glory and the dream: A narrative history of America.* New York: Bantam Books.

Meinert, R. (1998). Consequences for professional social work under conditions of postmodernity. *Social Thought,* 18(3):41-54.

Mullaly, B. (1997). *Structural social work: Ideology, theory, and practice,* New York: Oxford University Press.

Murphy, R. (1997). *Sociology and nature: Social action in context.* Boulder, CO: Westview Press.

Murphy, J. and Pardeck, T. (1998). Renewing social work practice through a postmodern perspective. *Social Thought,* 18(3):5-19.

Norris, C. (1993). *The truth about postmodernism.* Cambridge, MA: Blackwell Publishers.

Ohmae, K. (1995). *The end of the nation state: The rise of regional economies.* New York: The Free Press.

Pardeck, J., Murphy, J., and Chung, W.S. (1994). Social work and postmodernism. *Social Work and Social Sciences Review,* 5(2):113-123.

Payne, M. (1997). *Modern social work theory,* Second edition. Chicago: Lyceum Books, Inc.

Poster, M. (1995). *The second media age.* Cambridge, UK: Polity Press.

Reamer, F. (1993). *The philosophical foundations of social work.* New York: Columbia University Press.

Reisch, M. and Gambrill, E. (1997). *Social work in the 21st century.* Thousand Oaks, CA: Pine Forge Press.

Ritzer, G. (1992). *The McDonaldization of society.* London: Pine Force Press.

Saulnier, C. (1995). *Feminist theories and social work: Approaches and applications.* Binghamton, NY: The Haworth Press.

Soja, E. W. (1989). *Postmodern geographies: A reassertion of space in critical social theory.* New York: Verso Press.

Stoesz, D. (1997). The end of social work. In Reisch, M. and Gambrill, E. (Eds.), *Social work in the 21st century* (pp. 368-375). Thousand Oaks, CA: Pine Forge Press.

Stretch, J. (1967). Existentialism: A proposed philosophical orientation for social work. *Social Work,* 12(4):97-102.

Tenner, E. (1997). *Why things bite back: Technology and the revenge of unintended consequences.* New York: Random House.

Thurow, L. (1998). High-tech boom or productivity bust: Who knows? *USA Today,* Monday, March 9, 19A.

Tolson, E. (1988). *The metamodel and clinical social work.* New York: Columbia University Press.

Trattner, W. (1974). *From poor law to welfare state.* New York: The Free Press.

Turner, F. (1986). *Social work treatment: Interlocking theoretical approaches,* Third edition. Binghamton, NY: The Haworth Press.

Whelan, W. and Black, S. (1982). *From genetic experimentation to biotechnology —The critical transition.* New York: John Wiley and Sons.

Whittington, C. and Holland, R. (1985). A framework for theory in social work. *Issues in Social Work Education,* 5(1):25-50.

Wilensky, J. and Lebeaux, C. (1965). *Industrial society and social welfare.* New York: The Free Press.

Wise, J. (1997). *Exploring technology and social space.* Thousand Oaks, CA: Sage Publications.

Chapter 3

Abbott, A.A. (1985). Research productivity patterns of social work doctorates. *Social Work Research and Abstracts,* 21(3):11-17.

Brian, S. (1990). Empiricism and clinical practice. In Videka-Sherman, L. and Reid, W.J. (Eds.), *Advances in clinical social work research* (pp. 1-7). Silver Spring, MD: National Association of Social Workers.

Cheung, K.M. (1990). Interdisciplinary relationships between social work and other disciplines: A citation study. *Social Work Research and Abstracts,* 26(3):23-29.

Collins, R. (1975). *Conflict sociology: Toward an explanatory science.* New York: Academic Press.

Commission on Accreditation (1994). *Handbook of accreditation standards and procedures.* Washington, DC: Council on Social Work Education.

Epstein, W.M. (1990). Confirmation bias among social work journals. *Science, Technology, and Human Values,* 15(1):244-247.

Epstein, W.M. (1992). A response to Pardeck. Thump therapy for social work journals. *Research on Social Work Practice,* 2(4):525-528.

Fisher, D.V. (1991). *An introduction to constructivism for social work.* Westport, CT: Praeger.

Fraser, M.W., Lewis, R.E., and Norman, J.L. (1990). Research education in MSW programs: An exploratory analysis. *Journal of Teaching in Social Work,* 4(2): 83-103.

Fraser, M.W., Taylor, M.J., Jackson, R., and O'Jack, J. (1991). Social work and science: Many ways of knowing? *Social Work Research Abstracts,* 27(4):5-15.

Gingerich, W.J. (1990). Rethinking single-case evaluation. In Videka-Sherman, L. and Reid, W.J. (Eds.), *Advances in clinical social work research* (pp. 11-24). Silver Spring, MD: National Association of Social Workers.

Green, R.G., Hutchinson, E.D., and Sar, B.K. (1992). Evaluating scholarly performance: The productivity of graduates of social work doctoral programs. *Social Service Review,* 66(3):441-466.

Greenwood, E. (1957). Attributes of a profession. *Social Work,* 2(4):45-55.

Jenson, J.M., Fraser, M.W., and Lewis, R.E. (1991). Research training in social work doctoral programs. *Arete,* 16(1):23-38.

Kilpatrick, A.C. and Holland, T.P. (1995). *Working with families: An integrative model by level of functioning.* Boston: Allyn and Bacon.

Kirk, S.A. (1990). Research utilization: The substructure of belief. In Videka-Sherman, L. and Reid, W.J. (Eds.), *Advances in clinical social work research* (pp. 233-250). Silver Spring, MD: National Association of Social Workers.

Lindsey, D. (1976). Distinction, achievement, and editorial board membership. *American Psychologist,* 31(11):799-804.

Lindsey, D. (1977). Participation and influence in publication review proceedings: A reply. *American Psychologist,* 31(7):579-586.

Lindsey, D. (1999). Ensuring standards in social work research. *Research on Social Work Practice,* 9(1):115-120.

Mace, J.M. (1997). Introduction of chaos and complexity theory to social work. In Tucker, D.J., Garvin, C., and Sarri, R. (Eds.), *Integrating knowledge and practice* (pp. 149-158). Westport, CT: Praeger.

Midgley, J. (1999). Academic merit, professional needs, and social work education. *Research on Social Work Practice,* 9(1):104-107.

Pardeck, J. (1991). Using scientific practice increase scholarly activity among social work educators. *Education,* 111(2):382-387.

Pardeck, J. (1992a). Are social work editorial boards competent?: Some disquieting data with implications for social work practice. *Research on Social Work Practice,* 2(4):487-496.

Pardeck, J. (1992b). The distinction and achievement levels of social work editorial boards revisited. *Research on Social Work Practice, 2*(4):529-537.

Pardeck, J.T., Chung, W., and Murphy, J.W. (1997). Degreed and nondegreed licensed clinical social workers: An exploratory study. *Journal of Sociology and Social Welfare,* 24(2):143-158.

Pardeck, J.T. and Meinert, R. (1999). Scholarly achievements of the social work editorial board and consulting editors: A commentary. *Research on Social Work Practice,* 9(1):86-91.

Schilling, R.F. (1990). Making research usable. In Videka-Sherman, L. and Reid, W.I. (Eds.), *Advances in clinical social work research* (pp. 256-260). Silver Spring, MD: National Association of Social Workers.

Spaulding, E.C. (1991). *Statistics on social work education in the United States: 1990.* Alexandria, VA: Council on Social Work Education.

Thyer, B.A. (1997). Effective psychosocial treatments for children: A selective review. In Pardeck, J.T. and Markward, M. (Eds.), *Reassessing social work practice with children* (pp. 79-89). New York: Gordon and Breach.

U.S. Department of Education (1993). *Digest of education statistics.* National Center of Education Statistics. Washington, DC: U.S. Government Printing Office.

Chapter 4

Agger, B. (1991). *A critical theory of public life: Knowledge, discourse, and politics in an age of decline.* New York: The Falmer Press.

Agre, P. and Rotenberg, M. (1998). *Technology and privacy: The new landscape.* Cambridge, MA: MIT Press.

Biner, P.M. (1993). The development of an instrument to measure student attitudes towards televised courses. *American Journal of Distance Education,* 7(1):62-73.

Birkerts, S. (1996). The electronic hive. Refuse it. In Kling, R. (Ed.), *Computeriza tion and controversy: Value conflicts and social choice* (pp. 79-82). San Diego, CA: Academic Press.

Blakely, T.J. (1994). Strategies for distance learning. *Journal of Continuing Social Work Education,* 6(1):4-7.

Born, C. (1987). Microcomputers and field instruction. *Journal of Social Work Education,* 23(2):135-141.

Brindley L. (Ed.). (1989). *The electronic campus: An information strategy.* British Library: Boston Spa.

Brooks, M. (1997). Beyond teaching and learning: Trekking into the virtual university. *Teaching Sociology,* 25(1):1-14.

Caputo, R. (1991). Managing information systems: An ethical framework and information needs matrix. *Administration in Social Work,* 15(4):53-64.

Carey, J. (1991). Plato at the keyboard: Telecommunications technology and education policy. *The Annals of the American Academy of Political and Social Science,* 514 (March):11-21.

Cnaan, R. and Parsloe, P. (1989). *The impact of information technology on social work practice.* New York: The Haworth Press.

Conklin, J.J. and Osterndorf, W. (1995). Distance learning in continuing social work education: Promise of the year 2000. *Journal of Continuing Social Work Education,* 6(3):13-17.

Connick, G. (1997). Issues and trends to take us into the twenty-first century. In Cyrs, T. (Ed.), *Teaching and learning at a distance: What it takes to effectively design, deliver, and evaluate programs* (pp. 7-12). Evanston, IL: Jossey-Bass Publishers.

Cwikel, J. and Cnaan, R. (1991). Ethical dilemmas in applying second-wave information technology to social work practice. *Social Work,* 36(2):114-120.

Dede, C. (1991). Emerging technologies: Impacts on distance learning. *The Annals of the American Academy of Political and Social Science,* 514 (March):146-158.

Derrida, J. (1976). *Of grammatology,* translated by G.C. Spivak. Baltimore: The Johns Hopkins University Press.

Epstein, W. (1995). Social work in the university. *Journal of Social Work in Education,* 31(2):281-292.

Ferre, F. (1995). *Philosophy of technology.* Athens, GA: The University of Georgia Press.

Fisher, W. (1992). Narration, Reason and Community. In Brown, R.H. (Ed.), *Writing the social text: Poetics and politics in social science discourse* (pp. 199-219). New York: Aldine De Gruyter.

Fisher, W. (1995). The economic context of community-centered practice: Markets, communities, and social policy. In Adams, P. and Nelson, K. (Eds.), *Reinventing human services: Community and family-centered practice* (pp. 41-58). New York: Aldine De Gruyter.

Gandy, J. and Tepperman, L. (1990). *False alarm: The computerization of eight social welfare organizations.* Ontario, Canada: Wilfrid Laurier University Press.

Giddens, A. (1984). *The constitution of society: Outline of the theory of structuration.* Cambridge, England: Polity Press.

Giffords, E. (1998). Social work on the Internet: An introduction. *Social Work,* 43(3): 243-251.

Goffman, E. (1959). *The presentation of self in everyday life.* Garden City, NY: Doubleday Publishers.

Gottdiener, M. (1985). *The social production of urban space.* Austin, TX: University of Texas Press.

Hassan, I. (1982). *The dismemberment of Orpheus: Towards a postmodern literature.* New York: O.U. Publishers.

Hauerwas, S. and Jones, G. (1989). *Why narrative?: Readings in narrative theology.* Grand Rapids, MI: William B. Eerdmans Publishing Company.

Hawkins, J. (1991). Technology-mediated communities for learning: Designs and consequences. *The Annals of the American Academy of Political and Social Science,* 514 (March):159-174.

Howard, M. (1995). From oral tradition to computerization: A case study of a social work department. *Computers in Human Services,* 12(3-4):203-219.

Iacono, S. and Kling, R. (1996). Computerization, office routines, and changes in clerical work. In Kling, R. (Ed.), *Computerization and controversy: Value conflicts and social choices* (pp. 51-55). San Diego, CA: Academic Press.

Johnstone, S. (1991). Research on telecommunicated learning: Past, present and future. *The Annals of the American Academy of Political and Social Science,* 514 (March):49-57.

Jones, A., Kirkup, G., and Kirwood, A. (1993). *Personal computers for distance education: A study of an educational innovation.* New York: St. Martin's Press.

Karger, H. (1983). Science, research and social work: Or, who controls the profession and how? *Social Work,* 28(3):214-216.

Karger H. and Kreuger, L. (1988). Technology and the "not always so human" services. *Computers in Human Services,* 3(1):111-126.

Kling, R. (1996). *Computerization and controversy: Value conflicts and social choices.* San Diego, CA: Academic Press.

Kreuger, L. (1993). Should there be a moratorium on articles that rank schools of social work based on faculty publications? Yes! *Journal of Social Work Education,* 29(3):240-252.

Kreuger, L. (1997). The end of social work. *Journal of Social Work Education,* 33(1): 19-27.

Kubey, R. and Csikszentmihalyi, M. (1990). *Television and the quality of life: How viewing shapes everyday experience.* Hillsdale, NJ: Lawrence Erlbaum Associates.

LaMendola, W. (1987). Teaching information technology to social workers. *Journal of Teaching in Social Work,* 1(1):53-69.

Lynett, P. (1985). The current and potential uses of computer assisted interactive videodisc in education of social workers. *Computers in Human Services,* 1(4): 75-85.

Marcuse, H. (1964). *One dimensional man: Studies in the ideology of advanced industrial society.* Boston: Beacon Press.

McWilliam, E. and Taylor, P. (1996). *Pedagogy, technology, and the body.* New York: Peter Lang.

Memmott, J. and Brennan, E. (1998). Learner-learning environment fit: An adult learning model for social work education. *Journal of Teaching in Social Work,* 16(1/2):75-83.

Monnickendam, M. and Eaglestein, S. (1993). Computer acceptance by social workers: Some unexpected research findings. *Computer in Human Services,* 9(3-4):409-424.

O'Reilly, C. (1980). Individuals and information overload in organizations: Is more necessarily better? *Academy of Management Journal,* 23:684-696.

Orme, J.G. and Combs-Orme, T. (1986). Statistical power and type II errors in social work research. *Social Work Research and Abstracts,* 22(3):3-10.

Pardeck, J.T. (1992). Are social work journal editorial boards competent? Some disquieting data with implications for research on social work practice, *Research on Social Work Practice,* 2(4):487-496.

Patterson, D. and Yaffe, J. (1994). Hypermedia computer-based education in social work education. *Journal of Social Work Education,* 30(2):267-277.

Paul, R.H. (1990). *Open learning and open management: Leadership and integrity in distance education.* London: Kogan Page.

Perelman, L.J. (1992). *School's out: Hyperlearning, the new technology, and the end of education.* New York: William Morrow.

Phillips, D. and Berman, Y. (1997). *Human services in the age of new technology: Harmonizing social work and computerization.* Brookfield, VT: Ashgate Publishing Company.

Pickering, A. (1995). *The mangle of practice: Time, agency, and science.* Chicago: The University of Chicago Press.

Poster, M. (1990). *The mode of information: Poststructuralism and social context.* Chicago: The University of Chicago Press.

Reamer, F. (1986). The use of technology in social work: Ethical dilemmas. *Social Work,* 31(6):469-472.

Ritzer, G. (1992). *The McDonaldization of society.* London: Pine Force Press.

Saleebey, D. (1991). Technological fix: Altering the consciousness of the social work profession. *Journal of Sociology and Social Welfare,* 18(4):51-67.

Sassone, P. (1992). Survey finds low office productivity linked to staffing imbalances. *National Productivity Review,* 11(2):147-158.

Schopler, J., Abell, M., and Galinsky, M. (1998). Technology-based groups: A review and conceptual framework for practice. *Social Work,* 43(3):254-267.

Seabury, B. and Maple, F. (1993). Using computers to teach practice skills. *Social Work,* 38(4):430-439.

Siegel, E., Jennings, J., Conklin, J., and Flynn, S. (1998). Distance learning in social work education: Results and implications of a national survey. *Journal of Social Work Education,* 34(1):71-80.

Sproull, L. and Kiesler, S. (1996). Increasing personal connections. In Kling, R., *Computerization and controversy: Value conflicts and social choices* (pp. 455-475). San Diego, CA: Academic Press.

Stretch, J. (1967). Existentialism: A proposed philosophical orientation for social work. *Social Work,* 12(4):97-102.

Stretch, J. and Kreuger, L. (1992). New challenges of technology for social work administrators. In Healey, L. (Ed.), *Managers choices: Compelling issues in the new decision environment* (pp. 56-64). Washington, DC: NASW Publications.

Tenner, E. (1997). *Why things bite back: Technology and the revenge of unintended consequences.* New York: Random House.

Thurow, L. (1998). High-tech boom or productivity bust: Who knows? *USA Today,* Monday, March 9, 19A.

Thyer, B., Polk, G., and Gaudin, J. (1997). Distance learning in social work education: A preliminary evaluation. *Journal of Social Work Education,* 33(2):363-367.

Tufte, E. (1983). *The visual display of quantitative information.* Chesire, CT: Graphics Press.

Warf, B. (1991). Structuration theory and electronic communications. In Wilson, D. and Huff, J. (Eds.), *Marginalized Places and Populations: A Structuralist Agenda.* Westport, CT: Praeger.

Warriner-Burke, H. (1990). Distance learning: What we don't know won't hurt us. *Foreign Language Annals,* 23(2):129-133.

Wise, J.M. (1997). *Exploring technology and social space.* Thousand Oaks, CA: Sage Publications.

Wodarski, J. and Kelly, T. (1987). Simulation technology in social work education. *ARETE,* 12(2):12-20.

Zigerell, J. (1991). *The uses of television in American higher education.* New York: Praeger.

Chapter 5

Austin, D. (1997). The institutional development of social work education: The first 100 years—and beyond. *Journal of Social Work Education,* 33(3):599-612.

Bisno, H. and Cox, F. (1997). Social work education: Catching up with the present and future. *Journal of Social Work Education,* 33(2):373-387.

Brooks, V. (1982). Specializations: Current development and the myth of innovation. *Journal of Social Work Education,* 18(3):31-36.

CSWE (1992a). *Curriculum policy statement for baccalaureate degree programs in social work education.* Alexandria, VA: Council on Social Work Education.

CSWE (1992b). *Curriculum policy statement for master's degree programs in social work education.* Alexandria, VA: Council on Social Work Education..

CSWE (1994a). *Baccalaureate evaluative standards and interpretive guidelines.* Alexandria, VA: Council on Social Work Education.

CSWE (1994b). *Master's evaluative standards and interpretive guidelines.* Alexandria, VA: Council on Social Work Education.

CSWE (1997). *Statistics on social work education in the United States: 1997.* Alexandria, VA: Council on Social Work Education.

CSWE (1998). *Directory of colleges and universities with accredited social work degree programs.* Alexandria, VA: Council on Social Work Education.

Dinerman, M. (1994). Issues in social work education. In Meinert, R., Pardeck, J., and Sullivan, W. (Eds.), *Issues in social work: A critical analysis* (pp. 127-146). Westport, CT: Greenwood Press.

Flexner, A. (1915). Is social work a profession? *Proceedings of the National Conference of Charities and Corrections.* Chicago: Hildmann Printing, 576-590.

Gross, G. (1992). A defining moment: The social work continuum revisited. *Journal of Social Work Education,* 28(1):110-118.

Hartman, A. (1983). Concentrations, specializations, and curriculum design in MSW and BSW programs. *Journal of Social Work Education,* 19(2):16-25.

Hollis, E. and Taylor, A. (1951). *Social work education in the United States.* New York: Columbia University Press.

Kirk, S. and Corcoran, K. (1995). School rankings: Mindless narcissism or do they tell us something. *Journal of Social Work Education,* 31(3):408-414.

Koerner, B. (1998). Health disciplines: The top schools in the U.S. news surveys. *U.S. News and World Report,* 122(9) (March):88.

Kreuger, L. (1993). Should there be a moratorium on articles that rank schools of social work based on faculty publications? Yes! *Journal of Social Work Education,* 29(3):240-245.

Landon, P. (1995). Generalist and advanced generalist practice. In Edwards, R. (Ed.), *Encyclopedia of social work,* Nineteenth edition. Washington, DC: NASW Press.

Meinert, R. (1979). Concentrations: Empirical patterns and future prospects. *Journal of Social Work Education,* 15(2):51-58.

Meinert, R. (1993). Should there be a moratorium on articles that rank schools of social work based on faculty publications? No! *Journal of Social Work Education,* 29(3):245-251.

NASW (1974). Social case work generic and specific: A report of the Milford conference, 1929. Reprinted from *American Association of Social Workers.* New York: National Association of Social Workers.

Pardeck, J., Yuen, F., Daley, J., and Hawkins, C. (1998). Social work assessment and intervention through family health practice. *Family Therapy,* 25(1):25-39.

Raymond, G., Teare, R., and Atherton, C. (1996). Is "field of practice" a relevant organizing principle for the MSW curriculum? *Journal of Social Work Education,* 32(1):19-30.

Chapter 6

Adam, S. and Orgel, M. (1975). *Through the mental health maze: A consumer's guide to finding a psychotherapist.* Washington, DC: Health Research Group, Public Citizen.

Beck, A. (1976). *Cognitive therapy and emotional disorder.* New York: International Universities Press.

Berger, R.M. (1990). Getting published: A mentoring program for social work faculty. *Social Work,* 35:69-71.

Bloom, M. (1978). Challenges to helping professions and the response of scientific practice. *Social Service Review,* 52:584-595.

Briar, S. (1979). Incorporating research into education for clinical practice. In Rubin, A. and Rosenblatt, A. (Eds.), *Social work: Toward a clinical science in social work.* New York: Council on Social Work Education.

Campbell, J. (1988). Client acceptance of single-system evaluation. *Social Work Research and Abstracts,* 24(2):21-22.

Centra, J.A. (1979). *Determining faculty effectiveness.* San Francisco: Jossey-Bass.

Connaway, R. and Gentry, M. (1988). *Social work practice.* Englewood Cliffs, NJ: Prentice-Hall.

Council on Social Work Education (1994). *Handbook of accreditation standards and procedures.* Alexandria, VA: Council on Social Work Education.

Dinerman, M. (1981). *Social work curriculum at baccalaureate and masters level.* New York: The Lois and Samuel Silberman Fund.

Ellis, A. (1997). Extending the goals of behavior and cognitive behavioral therapy. *Behavior Therapy,* 28(3):333-339.

Euster, G. and Weinbach, R. (1986). Deans' quality assessment of faculty publications for tenure/promotion decisions. *Journal of Social Work Education,* 22(3): 79-84.

Fraser, M.W. (1994). Scholarship and research in social work: Emerging challenges. *Journal of Social Work Education,* 30(2):252-266.

Fraser, M.W., Lewis, R.E., and Norman, J.L. (1990). Research education in MSW programs: An exploratory analysis. *Journal of Teaching in Social Work,* 4(2): 83-103.

Glasser, W. (1969). *The identity society.* New York: Harper and Row.

Green, R.G., Hutchinson, E.D., and Sar, B.K. (1992). Evaluating scholarly performance: The productivity of graduates of social work doctoral programs. *Social Service Review,* 66(3):441-446.

Grinnell, R., Kyte, N., and Hunter, M. (1979). The research component of doctoral programs in social work: A survey. *Journal of Sociology and Social Welfare,* 6(3):375-384.

Hudson, W.W. (1984). Indexes and scales. In Grinnell, R.M. (Ed.), *Social work research and evaluation.* Homewood, IL: Dorsey Press.

Krumboltz, J. (1966). Behavioral counseling. *Journal of Counseling Psychology,* 13(2):153-159.

Krumboltz, J. and Hosford, R. (1967). Behavioral counseling in the elementary school. *Elementary School Guidance and Counseling,* 1:27-40.

Lindsey, D. (1976). Distinction, achievement, and editoral board membership. *American Psychologist,* 31(11):799-804.

NASW (1996). *Code of Ethics.* Washington, DC: National Association of Social workers.

Pardeck, J.T. (1991). Using scientific practice to increase scholarly activity among social work educators. *Education,* 111(2):195-199.

Pardeck, J.T. (1994). *Using bibliotherapy in clinical practice: A guide to self-help books.* Westport, CT: Greenwood Press.

Pardeck, J.T. (1996). *Social work practice: An ecological approach.* Westport, CT: Auburn House.

Pardeck, J.T. and Murphy, J. (1986). Technology and the therapeutic relationship. *Family Therapy* (Special Issue), 16.

Pardeck, J.T. and Pardeck, J.A. (1987). Using bibliotherapy to help children cope with the changing family. *Social Work in Education,* 9(2):107-116.

Sagan, C. (1997). *The demon-haunted world: Science as a candle in the dark.* New York: Ballantine Books.

Schilling, R.F., Schinke, S.P., and Gilchrist, L.D. (1985). Utilization of social work research: Reaching the practitioner. *Social Work,* 30(6):527-529.

Sheafor, B.W., Hurejsi, G.P., and Hurejsi, G.A. (1988). *Techniques and guidelines for social work practice.* Boston: Allyn and Bacon.

Siporin, M. (1975). *Introduction to social work practice.* New York: Macmillan.

Skinner, B.F. (1953). *Science and human behavior.* New York: Macmillan.

Spaulding, E.C. (1991). *Statistics on social work education in the United States: 1990.* Alexandria, VA: Council on Social Work Education.

Task Force on Social Work Research (1991). *Building social work knowledge for effective services and policies: A plan for research development.* Austin, TX: Capital Printing.

Thomas, E.J. (1977). The BESDAS model for effective practice. *Social Work Research and Abstracts,* 13(2):12-16.

Thompson, C.L. and Rudolph, L.B. (1992). *Counseling children,* Third edition. Pacific Grove, CA: Brooks/Cole.

Thyer, B.A. (1997). Effective psychosocial treatments for children: A selective review. In Pardeck, J.T. and Markward, M. (Eds.), *Reassessing social work practice with children* (pp. 79-89). New York: Gordon and Breach.

Van Houten, R., Axelrod, S., Bailey, J.S., Favell, J.E., Foxx, R.M., Iwata, B.A., and Lovaas, O.J. (1988). The right to effective behavioral treatment. *The Behavior Analyst,* 11(2):111-114.

Index

HAWORTH Social Work Practice in Action
Carlton E. Munson, PhD, Senior Editor

HUMAN SERVICES AND THE AFROCENTRIC PARADIGM by Jerome H. Schiele. (2000). "Represents a milestone in applying the Afrocentric paradigm to human services generally, and social work specifically. . . . A highly valuable resource." *Bogart R. Leashore, PhD, Dean and Professor, Hunter College School of Social Work, New York, New York*

SOCIAL WORK: SEEKING RELEVANCY IN THE TWENTY-FIRST CENTURY by Roland Meinert, John T. Pardeck and Larry Kreuger. (2000). "Highly recommended. A thought-provoking work that asks the difficult questions and challenges the status quo. A great book for graduate students as well as experienced social workers and educators." *Francis K. O. Yuen, DSW, ACSE, Associate Professor, Division of Social Work, California State University, Sacramento*

SOCIAL WORK PRACTICE IN HOME HEALTH CARE by Ruth Ann Goode. (2000). "Dr. Goode presents both a lucid scenario and a formulated protocol to bring health care services into the home setting. . . . This is a must have volume that will be a reference to be consulted many times." *Marcia B. Steinhauer, PhD, Coordinator and Associate Professor, Human Services Administration Program, Rider University, Lawrenceville, New Jersey*

FORENSIC SOCIAL WORK: LEGAL ASPECTS OF PROFESSIONAL PRACTICE, SECOND EDITION by Robert L. Barker and Douglas M. Branson. (2000). "The authors combine their expertise to create this informative guide to address legal practice issues facing social workers." *Newsletter of the National Organization of Forensic Social Work*

SOCIAL WORK IN THE HEALTH FIELD: A CARE PERSPECTIVE by Lois A. Fort Cowles. (1999). "Makes an important contribution to the field by locating the practice of social work in health care within an organizational and social context." *Goldie Kadushin, PhD, Associate Professor, School of Social Welfare, University of Wisconsin, Milwaukee*

SMART BUT STUCK: WHAT EVERY THERAPIST NEEDS TO KNOW ABOUT LEARNING DISABILITIES AND IMPRISONED INTELLIGENCE by Myrna Orenstein. (1999). "A trailblazing effort that creates an entirely novel way of talking and thinking about learning disabilities. There is simply nothing like it in the field." *Fred M. Levin, MD, Training Supervising Analyst, Chicago Institute for Psychoanalysis; Assistant Professor of Clinical Psychiatry, Northwestern University, School of Medicine, Chicago, IL*

CLINICAL WORK AND SOCIAL ACTION: AN INTEGRATIVE APPROACH by Jerome Sachs and Fred Newdom. (1999). "Just in time for the new millennium come Sachs and Newdom with a wholly fresh look at social work. . . . A much-needed uniting of social work values, theories, and practice for action." *Josephine Nieves, MSW, PhD, Executive Director, National Association of Social Workers*

SOCIAL WORK PRACTICE IN THE MILITARY by James G. Daley. (1999). "A significant and worthwhile book with provocative and stimulating ideas. It deserves to be read by a wide audience in social work education and practice as well as by decision makers in the military." *H. Wayne Johnson, MSW, Professor, University of Iowa, School of Social Work, Iowa City, Iowa*

GROUP WORK: SKILLS AND STRATEGIES FOR EFFECTIVE INTERVEN-TIONS, SECOND EDITION by Sondra Brandler and Camille P. Roman. (1999). "A clear, basic description of what group work requires, including what skills and techniques group workers need to be effective." *Hospital and Community Psychiatry* (from the first edition)

TEENAGE RUNAWAYS: BROKEN HEARTS AND "BAD ATTITUDES" by Laurie Schaffner (1999). "Skillfully combines the authentic voice of the juvenile runaway with the principles of social science research."

CELEBRATING DIVERSITY: COEXISTING IN A MULTICULTURAL SOCIETY by Benyamin Chetkow-Yanoov. (1999). "Makes a valuable contribution to peace theory and practice." *Ian Harris, EdD, Executive Secretary, Peace Education Committee, International Peace Research Association*

SOCIAL WELFARE POLICY ANALYSIS AND CHOICES by Hobart A. Burch. (1999). "Will become the landmark text in its field for many decades to come." *Sheldon Rahan, DSW, Founding Dean and Emeritus Professor of Social Policy and Social Administration. Faculty of Social Work, Wilfrid Laurier University, Canada*

SOCIAL WORK PRACTICE: A SYSTEMS APPROACH, SECOND EDITION by Benyamin Chetkow-Yannov. (1999). "Highly recommended as a primary text for any and all introductory social work courses." *Ram A. Cnaan, PhD, Associate Professor, School of Social Work, University of Pennsylvania*

CRITICAL SOCIAL WELFARE ISSUES: TOOLS FOR SOCIAL WORK AND HEALTH CARE PROFESSIONALS edited by Arthur J. Katz, Abraham Lurie, and Carlos M. Vidal. (1997). "Offers hopeful agendas for change, while navigating the societal challenges facing those in the human services today." *Book News Inc.*

SOCIAL WORK IN HEALTH SETTINGS: PRACTICE IN CONTEXT, SECOND EDITION edited by Toba Schwaber Kerson. (1997). "A first-class document . . . It will be found among the steadier and lasting works on the social work aspects of American health care." *Hans S. Falck, PhD, Professor Emeritus and Former Chair, Health Specialization in Social Work, Virginia Commonwealth University*

PRINCIPLES OF SOCIAL WORK PRACTICE: A GENERIC PRACTICE APPROACH by Molly R. Hancock. (1997). "Hancock's discussions advocate reflection and self-awareness to create a climate for client change." *Journal of Social Work Education*

NOBODY'S CHILDREN: ORPHANS OF THE HIV EPIDEMIC by Steven F. Dansky. (1997). "Professional sound, moving, and useful for both professionals and interested readers alike." *Ellen G. Friedman, ACSW, Associate Director of Support Services, Beth Israel Medical Center, Methadone Maintenance Treatment Program*

SOCIAL WORK APPROACHES TO CONFLICT RESOLUTION: MAKING FIGHTING OBSOLETE by Benyamin Chetkow-Yanoov. (1996). "Presents an examination of the nature and cause of conflict and suggests techniques for coping with conflict." *Journal of Criminal Justice*

FEMINIST THEORIES AND SOCIAL WORK: APPROACHES AND APPLICATIONS by Christine Flynn Salunier. (1996). " An essential reference to be read repeatedly by all educators and practitioners who are eager to learn more about feminist theory and practice: *Nancy R. Hooyman, PhD, Dean and Professor, School of Social Work, University of Washington, Seattle*

THE RELATIONAL SYSTEMS MODEL FOR FAMILY THERAPY: LIVING IN THE FOUR REALITIES by Donald R. Bardill. (1996). "Engages the reader in quiet, thoughtful conversation on the timeless issue of helping families and individuals." *Christian Counseling Resource Review*

SOCIAL WORK INTERVENTION IN AN ECONOMIC CRISIS: THE RIVER COMMUNITIES PROJECT by Martha Baum and Pamela Twiss. (1996). "Sets a standard for universities in terms of the types of meaningful roles they can play in supporting and sustaining communities." *Kenneth J. Jaros, PhD, Director, Public Health Social Work Training Program, University of Pittsburgh*

FUNDAMENTALS OF COGNITIVE-BEHAVIOR THERAPY: FROM BOTH SIDES OF THE DESK by Bill Borcherdt. (1996). "Both beginning and experienced practitioners . . . will find a considerable number of valuable suggestions in Borcherdt's book." *Albert Ellis, PhD, President, Institute for Rational-Emotive Therapy, New York City*

BASIC SOCIAL POLICY AND PLANNING: STRATEGIES AND PRACTICE METHODS by Hobart A. Burch. (1996). "Burch's familiarity with his topic is evident and his book is an easy introduction to the field." *Readings*

THE CROSS-CULTURAL PRACTICE OF CLINICAL CASE MANAGEMENT IN MENTAL HEALTH edited by Peter Manoleas. (1996). "Makes a contribution by bringing together the cross-cultural and clinical case management perspectives in working with those who have serious mental illness." *Disability Studies Quarterly*

FAMILY BEYOND FAMILY: THE SURROGATE PARENT IN SCHOOLS AND OTHER COMMUNITY AGENCIES by Sanford Weinstein. (1995). "Highly recommended to anyone concerned about the welfare of our children and the breakdown of the American family." *Jerold S. Greenberg, EdD, Director of Community Service, College of Health & Human Performance, University of Maryland*

PEOPLE WITH HIV AND THOSE WHO HELP THEM: CHALLENGES, INTEGRATION, INTERVENTION by R. Dennis Shelby. (1995). "A useful and compassionate contribution to the HIV psychotherapy literature." *Public Health*

THE BLACK ELDERLY: SATISFACTION AND QUALITY OF LATER LIFE by Marguerite Coke and James A. Twaite. (1995). "Presents a model for predicting life satisfaction in this population." *Abstracts in Social Gerontology*

BUILDING ON WOMEN'S STRENGTHS: A SOCIAL WORK AGENDA FOR THE TWENTY-FIRST CENTURY edited by Liane V. Davis. (1994). "The most lucid and accessible overview of the related epistemological debates int he social work literature." *Journal of the National Association of Social Workers*

NOW DARE EVERYTHING: TALES OF HIV-RELATED PSYCHOTHERAPY by Steven F. Dansky. (1994). "A highly recommended book for anyone working with persons who are HIV positive. . . . Every library should have a copy of this book." *AIDS Book Review Journal*

INTERVENTION RESEARCH: DESIGN AND DEVELOPMENT FOR HUMAN SERVICE edited by Jack Rothman and Edwin J. Thomas. (1994). "Provides a useful framework for the further examination of methodology for each separate step of such research." *Academic Library Book Review*

CLINICAL SOCIAL WORK SUPERVISION, SECOND EDITION by Carlton E. Munson. (1993). "A useful, thorough, and articulate reference for supervisors and for 'supervisees' who are wanting to understand their supervisor or are looking for effective supervision." *Transactional Analysis Journal*

ELEMENTS OF THE HELPING PROCESS: A GUIDE FOR CLINICIANS by Raymond Fox. (1993). "Filled with helpful hints, creative interventions, and practical guidelines." *Journal of Family Psychotherapy*

IF A PARTNER HAS AIDS: GUIDE TO CLINICAL INTERVENTION FOR RELATIONSHIPS IN CRISIS by R. Dennis Shelby. (1993). " A welcome addition to existing publications about couples coping with AIDS, it offers intervention ideas and strategies to clinicians." *Contemporary Psychology*

GERONTOLOGICAL SOCIAL WORK SUPERVISION by Ann Burack-Weiss and Frances Coyle Brennan. (1991). "The creative ideas in this book will aid supervisors working with students and experienced social workers." *Senior News*

SOCIAL WORK THEORY AND PRACTICE WITH THE TERMINALLY ILL by Joan K. Parry. (1989). "Should be read by all professionals engaged in the provision of health services in hospitals, emergency rooms, and hospices." *Hector B. Garcia, PhD, Professor, San Jose State University School of Social Work*

THE CREATIVE PRACTITIONER: THEORY AND METHODS FOR THE HELPING SERVICES by Bernard Gelfand. (1988). "[Should] be widely adopted by those in the helping services. It could lead to significant positive advances by countless individuals." *Sidney J. Parnes, Trustee Chairperson for Strategic Program Development, Creative Education Foundation, Buffalo, NY*

MANAGEMENT AND INFORMATION SYSTEMS IN HUMAN SERVICES: IMPLICATIONS FOR THE DISTRIBUTION OF AUTHORITY AND DECISION MAKING by Richard K. Caputo. (1987). "A contribution to social work scholarship in that it provides conceptual frameworks that can be used in the design of management information systems." *Social Work*

Order Your Own Copy of
This Important Book for Your Personal Library!

SOCIAL WORK
Seeking Relevancy in the Twenty-First Century

_____ in hardbound at $39.95 (ISBN: 0-7890-0644-8)

_____ in softbound at $24.95 (ISBN: 0-7890-1050-X)

COST OF BOOKS_____

OUTSIDE USA/CANADA/
MEXICO: ADD 20%_____

POSTAGE & HANDLING_____
*(US: $3.00 for first book & $1.25
for each additional book)
Outside US: $4.75 for first book
& $1.75 for each additional book)*

SUBTOTAL_____

IN CANADA: ADD 7% GST_____

STATE TAX_____
*(NY, OH & MN residents, please
add appropriate local sales tax)*

FINAL TOTAL_____
*(If paying in Canadian funds,
convert using the current
exchange rate. UNESCO
coupons welcome.)*

☐ **BILL ME LATER:** ($5 service charge will be added)
(Bill-me option is good on US/Canada/Mexico orders only;
not good to jobbers, wholesalers, or subscription agencies.)

☐ Check here if billing address is different from
shipping address and attach purchase order and
billing address information.

Signature_____

☐ **PAYMENT ENCLOSED: $_____**

☐ **PLEASE CHARGE TO MY CREDIT CARD.**

☐ Visa ☐ MasterCard ☐ AmEx ☐ Discover
☐ Diners Club
Account #_____   _____

Exp. Date_____

Signature_____

Prices in US dollars and subject to change without notice.

NAME _____

INSTITUTION _____

ADDRESS _____

CITY _____

STATE/ZIP _____

COUNTRY _____ COUNTY (NY residents only) _____

TEL _____ FAX _____

E-MAIL_____
May we use your e-mail address for confirmations and other types of information? ☐ Yes ☐ No

Order From Your Local Bookstore or Directly From
The Haworth Press, Inc.
10 Alice Street, Binghamton, New York 13904-1580 • USA
TELEPHONE: 1-800-HAWORTH (1-800-429-6784) / Outside US/Canada: (607) 722-5857
FAX: 1-800-895-0582 / Outside US/Canada: (607) 772 6362
E-mail: getinfo@haworthpressinc.com
PLEASE PHOTOCOPY THIS FORM FOR YOUR PERSONAL USE.

BOF96